I Do Like To Be Beside The Seaside

To R.o.b

Love

Nettie

x

I Do Like To Be Beside The Seaside

Maria de la Mann

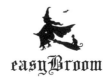

easyBroom

I Do Like To Be Beside The Seaside

An easyBroom book

Copyright © 2023 Maria de la Mann

ISBN 978-0957628878

The right of Maria de la Mann to be identified as the author of this work has been asserted in accordance with sections 77 and 78 of the Copyright, Designs and Patents Act 1988

Front cover photograph by Nigel Harpur. Back cover photograph, illustrations and cover design: Maria de la Mann

A catalogue record of this book is available from
The British Library

Books by the author

Verity Red's Diary (A story of surviving M.E.)

Love & Best Witches

Verity Writes Again

Verity Red (part one)

Verity Red (part two)

Verity Red (part three)

Is this really happening?

mariadelamann.co.uk

for Julia & Paul

Dedicated to the memory of

Jerry's wife Elizabeth

Acknowledgements

Thank you very much once again to Julia for her fabulous proof reading. I can hear myself saying, *'Oh, how did I miss that? How on earth did I miss that?'*

A whole book full of thank yous to my partner Nigel for a great job helping me put *another* book together, assisting with the research, and making the whole self-publishing process a pleasure.

Cheers to Bill, Dave and Nigel for doing a wonderful job painting and decorating the beach hut. Their hard work was *most appreciated.*

Last but not least to my cats, Diamanda and Lovely for inspiration, dear little paws plodding on my laptop keys to improve my writing and endless, warm furry love.

Prologue

Verity Red has admired beach huts along the Kent coast for as long as she can remember.

Unable to afford one, instead, over the years she has collected artwork, bed linen, towels and fridge magnets featuring beach hut designs.

Creating a small, model beach on a shelf in her bathroom with sand, shells, a miniature deckchair, bucket and spade, and a beach ball; the main feature was a blue and white wooden – yes you guessed!

Will Verity realise her dream and find happiness in the place where she most likes to be, beside the seaside, beside the sea?

Read on....

Chapter One

April

Wednesday 27th

11.21 a.m.

BEN: Oh. It's a bit breezy.

ME: A bit breezy?! *A bit breezy!?!?* Are you joking? It's flippin' arctic, freeze you to the bone, blow you away, gale force something – probably nine – *very strong winds* from the North Sea.

BEN: Yes dear.

ME: I saw little arrows flying across the weather girl's map this morning, zooming into this coastline. In fact, I'll swear one of them was stabbing *right* where we are now.

BEN: You may be right. I should have parked the car nearer the path down the hill.

ME: Or what Ordnance Survey maps call the path on the coastal slope.

BEN: Yes, little Miss Cartographer.

ME: I think I must be a little Miss Crazy. Has it finally happened? Have I lost my tiny mind? Here I am at the seaside. Icy cold winds. And although I've wrapped up well – well I thought I had – I'm going to turn into an ice cube at any moment. And I'm going to look at beach huts, with the intention of buying one.

BEN: It'll be less breezy – I mean gale force something, icy winds from the North Sea, when we go down the hill – I mean, coastal slope.

11.23 a.m.

ME: Ah, yes. That's a bit better, now we have our backs to the wind.

BEN: Onwards and downwards to beach hut city.

ME: I didn't realise there were so many beach huts in Herne Bay. I love all the rainbow and ice cream colours, some stripy, some not. They bring to mind a neat row of colourful books on a bookshelf, don't you think?

BEN: If you say so dear.

ME: They look so silent and peaceful, staring out to sea.

BEN: Are you moved to poetry?

ME: My brain is too frozen at the moment – my little Miss Crazy brain, wanting to buy a beach hut. It was the coldest August on record a few years ago. Last October was the wettest. Today is November-ish, instead of April-ish. We could be heading for the coldest, wettest summer on record.

BEN: Or the hottest.

ME: Yes. Climate change is worrying. Am I making a bad decision?

BEN: No. You've always loved beach huts, haven't you.

ME: True.

BEN: Our house is full of beach hut themed things. Towels, bedding and fridge magnets.

ME: Wall hooks, cushion cover, beach hut solar powered lights. My little hut scene I created in the bathroom with a model beach hut, sand, pebbles and shells, miniature deckchair and a beach ball.

BEN: Tiny bucket and spade, plastic sandals and a lilo (laughing).

ME: Yes!

BEN: Now you have a little inheritance you can spend some of it making your dream come true. *And* the beach is your favourite place to be.

ME: We both like to be beside the seaside.

BEN: Yes, we do like to be beside the sea.... Are you going to burst into song?

ME: Not today. Where's the hut you saw on the internet?

BEN: We're here.

ME: Oh. Very nice. I like the bubblegum pink and white stripes. Looks freshly painted.

BEN: It's been refurbished inside too.

ME: I remember the photo you showed me online, the interior looked clean with lots of useful cupboards.

BEN: I haven't had a reply from the owner. So lets go and have a look at another one I saw with a *FOR SALE* notice on the back wall, when I came down here last week.

ME: Is it far?

BEN: About fifteen huts down.

11.28 a.m. The tide is coming in. Waves are crashing on the shore as we crunch our way along the pebbles. Then we crunch a little more..... until Ben stops.

BEN: Here we are.

ME: I like it... But it does look rundown and neglected. Sad, peeling, dark blue paintwork. Rusty metal bits. Broken banister. I love the faded yellow sun design on the roof though... I think the hut needs rescuing.

BEN: You and your rescuing. People, plants, creepy-crawlies, stray cats and now beach huts.

ME: I've a feeling a spiritual, artistic person resided here. I feel *drawn* to it!.... Did you call the owner?

BEN: I rang the contact number and spoke to the man who runs The Beach Hut Association. He said (patting peeling white paintwork on the banister) it's reduced in price a lot because of the condition it's in and the owner is keen to sell.

ME: Oh good. I think if I buy it I will keep the sunshine design. It could be a radiant yellow and the whole hut a beautiful vibrant, summer sky blue.

BEN: And a few white seagulls too (laughing).

ME: Maybe (smiling and shivering).

BEN: Shall we head back to the car now?

ME: Yes. Before I die of exposure!

11.39 a.m.   We defrost nicely on the journey home, in our comfortable, warm car.

ME: I think I'd like to buy the blue hut. Could you and Bill paint it and sort the rusty bits?

BEN: Yeah, no problem.

ME: That would be wonderful. Are there toilet facilities nearby, do you know?

BEN: No idea. I'll ask the Beach Hut Association chap – there might be some at the angler's club. That's not far.

ME: I noticed the building, about twenty huts away.

BEN: If not, I did have a look on the internet. You can get a porta-loo called a Kampa Khazi portable toilet. It gets great reviews from campers.

ME: Good name (giggling).

BEN: Looks like a pedal bin. There's an inner bucket you can take out. Most of the others advertised look like toilets..... It's a good price too.

ME: I'll keep it in mind. The old bladder isn't as strong as it used to be. And I don't want to be plodding a long way when I need *to go,* and by the time I've *been*, it won't be long before I've got to plod back again.

BEN: You do like your minty tea and decaf coffee.

ME: That I do. What about heating? I'd like to spend time at the hut on a chilly summer's or springtime day. Maybe early autumn days too.

BEN: To get electricity you can have a biggish, not huge, battery and a thing called an inverter. Would mean you can have a fan heater and whatever else, rather than a gas heater which can be prone to condensation.

ME: Sounds lovely. And it'll be great if you and Bill can make me interior doors with windows?

BEN: Yeah, we could do that.

ME: That would be brilliant! I've a joke for you.... A house went to the doctor and said – Doctor, doctor, I've got window pains. The doctor replied – Solar power is the future but it won't happen overnight.

WE LAUGH

Thursday 28th

BEN: I had another chat with Andrew.

ME: Andrew?

BEN: The man who runs the Herne Bay Beach Hut Association – nearly all sales go through them. I told him you were interested in the hut and he suggested I email him and he'll forward it to the owner. He said there will be a council rent and insurance to pay.

ME: Okay, I was expecting that.

BEN: Oh, and he said the Herne hutters –

ME: Herne nutters?!

BEN: Herne *hutters*. That's what they call themselves.

ME: I like that. Instead of a little nutter, I could be a little Herne hutter, who likes to eat fresh bread and butter.

BEN: Do you feel some verse coming on?

ME: Maybe...... What rhymes with hutter?..... flutter..... shutter....

BEN: Cheese cutter... for the cheese on bread and butter.

ME: Stutter.... mutter..... I don't feel inspired.

3.55 p.m. I head to the kitchen to switch the kettle on for a decaf coffee and digestive biscuit or two, to go with a delicious episode of *Château DIY*. Today at Château de Seguenville, Becky and Mark embark on their own huge gîte project. The floor has to be dug out, but the digger can't even fit through the entrance. I do love a bit of DIY in France – and it's entertaining when they run into difficulties.

3.56 p.m. I notice we've run out of decaf coffee and there's no fresh pack in the cupboard. But there is a lovely, new pack of minty tea in a pretty green box. I mutter to myself about my bad memory. But feel inspired.

The hutter was a nutter
Who would sit and quietly mutter

BEN: *She enjoyed fresh bread and butter*

ME: *And loved a French green shutter*

BEN: *He liked a good cheese cutter*

ME: Now I fancy some French cheese.

BEN: I'm popping down to Sainsbury's in a minute. I'll get coffee and eggs. Fresh loaf? French cheese?

ME: Oh, yes please!

BEN: About the Herne hutters – Andrew said they think their stretch of coast has a big advantage over Whitstable and Tankerton.

ME: Really? Why's that?

BEN: People walk in front of huts and peer in at you in Whitstable and Tankerton. The Herne Bay huts are right on the pebbly beach. Pebbles can be tiring to walk on, so most people use the path behind.

ME: That's not surprising. I remember when we went to look at the huts, people were walking their dogs on the path, not the pebbles. And it's good to see cycling is not allowed on the path.

BEN: Yeah.

ME: I'm starting to get a little excited now!

Friday 29th

1.10 p.m.

ME: This *Caprice des Dieux – un amour de fromage* is a very tasty cheese. Reminds me of Camembert. It's rich, soft and creamy. But creamier than Camembert. Heavenly.

BEN: That's probably why there are happy angels on the packaging.

ME: Oui. Ange parfait.

4.20 p.m.   I'm curled up with Diamanda, gently stroking her soft, black coat and warm, rose petal ears, while sipping a hot decaf coffee and watching *Château DIY* on Channel 4. Today Lee installs beams for the upper floor in the new two-bed gîte at Château Mareuil. The black cat winding around Lee's wife's legs, as she up-cycles a chest of drawers with a shabby chic look, makes me smile. The white cockatoo perched on their son's shoulder as he works on the château's grounds is charming, so is the little black dog, galloping around the grounds wearing a smart yellow rain jacket with a hood. But I can't help feeling a touch of envy, watching the big oak beams being installed. I like beams. Wooden rafters in my hut would suit me fine though.

ME: I hope there will be rafters in the blue hut, like we saw in the photos of the interior of the pink and white one.

BEN: I expect so.

ME: I could hang seasidey things from them.

BEN: And knowing you, my little witch, there will be a bat ornament or two.

ME: Of course. Although I'd prefer real bats. Like the ones I saw sleeping in the roof of a mill house where I used to stay in Bantry Bay, on the West Coast of Ireland.

BEN: Perhaps I can persuade a couple of bats to come to Herne Bay with us, from the group that fly around our sycamore tree at the bottom of the garden.

5.20 p.m.

BEN: I've just got a reply from Andrew about the hut. He says it's been closed up for a few years since the owner's wife passed away. It's full of loungers, tables and all sorts. And there's a kitchen unit, full of kitchen stuff that has seen better days. Oh, and there's a kayak that the owner says he hasn't got round to selling yet.

ME: The poor chap probably hasn't been able to face going back to the hut, it's so full of memories.

BEN: Yeah. I said we'd be happy to sell it for him.

ME: Oh good. But how will we transport a big, bloomin' kayak?

BEN: Bill's brother-in-law has a roof rack we could borrow. We used it when I helped Bill move house.

ME: That's handy. What about storage before we sell it?

BEN:	Bill or Rob.
ME:	Great!

8.23 p.m.   I'm watching *Midsomer Murders* with Lovely, my beautiful Persian blue, purring away on my lap (a purr as big as her heavy, warm body) as I stroke her soft head. We are glued to the TV. A wealthy land-owner's body has gone missing. DCI Barnaby, DS Nelson and new pathologist Kam Karimore investigate, and are drawn into the macabre world of body-snatching. Lovely flexes her claws and twitches her tail. Then widens her eyes. She seems to love a good murder/mystery.

ME: The beach hut is probably going to be full of rusty, musty, mouldy things. Mildew covered kitchen things. Loungers and windbreaks full of creepy-crawlies and spider webs. The life jackets could be rotting and there may be rotting wetsuits – the whole hut smelling like there's some sort of dead creature lurking in a corner. Or a dead body.

BEN: You've been watching too many episodes of *Midsomer Murders* and *Agatha Christie's Marple* dear.

ME: I must admit I've been watching more murder/mystery since you started spending more time at home.

WE LAUGH

Saturday 30th

7.23 p.m.   I'm engrossed in *Midsomer Murders* again, with Lovely. She's bored with this episode, yawns and falls asleep. We've probably seen it before and she knows the ending, but I don't remember. A pub land-lady is killed by an illusionist and pathologist Kate discovers sabotage is the cause. An evangelising curate claims the tragedy is God's vengeance for the pagan traditions held in Midsomer Oaks, but DCI Barnaby fears the illusionist was the real target.

ME: I think we should see inside the hut before I buy it, to see what condition it's in. You wouldn't buy a house before viewing inside would you. It gave the illusion of just needing a lick of paint and the rust sorted, but I think there could be hidden problems.

BEN: I showed Bill the photos I took of the roof and he said it looked okay. If there's a problem he knows how to repair roofing felt, he's done it before.

ME: That's good to know. The roof was one of my first concerns, would there be any holes in it.

There are holes in the sky
Where the rain gets in
But they're ever so small
That's why rain is thin

BEN: Very good (laughing).

ME: Yes, but I can't take the credit. It was written by the late, lovely Spike Milligan.

ME: Do you know when the hut owner will be back from his holiday?

BEN: Next weekend. I'll go down to the hut next weekend

to meet Andrew. He'll have the keys. I'll pick up Bill from Hastings and we can check out the hut together, it'll save you freezing and getting a chill again.

ME: That will be splendid (sniffling, followed by a big yawn), early night tonight I think.

BEN: Not slept much?

ME: I was woken up with nightmares. We were homeless and had to live in my beach hut, which was cold, and the walls covered in mould. It rained endlessly and the roof leaked onto a slimy, swirly green and brown seaweed covered floor. The rust on the door hinges became so bad that the doors fell off, letting freezing winds in and I could see giant, white arrows, like the ones on the weather girl's map after the news, flying across purple and yellow storm clouds, in our direction. The tide was in and huge waves splashed so close to the hut that we could feel sea spray on our faces. I'm shivering at the memory.

BEN: I'll turn the heating on. I'm sure you'll be havin' lovely dreams about happy beach huts after Bill and I have checked out the hut.

ME: I'm sure I will!

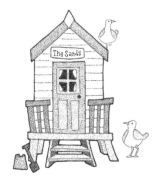

May

Sunday 1st

9.07 a.m.

ME: What's up? Headache?

BEN: Yeah. And we've run out of ibuprofen.

ME: Wanda of Weekly Witch said the other day, peppermint works faster on soothing a headache than pain killers. I have some minty aromatherapy oil somewhere in the bathroom cabinet. She also said the scent of an apple has good pain killing properties too. So here's a nice, fresh apple, have a good old sniff and I'll find the minty oil.

BEN: Anything you say dear.

9.10 a.m.

ME: Better?

BEN: Yeah. Surprisingly.

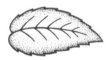

ME: I know I haven't bought the hut yet. Nothing agreed. Nothing signed. But I've been thinking about the shade of blue and yellow I'd like it painted.

BEN: That *doesn't* surprise me.

ME: I'd like a cheerful blue instead of the sad, dark blue it is the moment. A little like this turquoise tee-shirt. Or a bit darker, like this envelope folder. I spotted a lovely blue in TV Weekly – I'll have to find the page. Oh, and look at the light blue on our cushion with cat designs. Nice isn't it.

BEN: I think my headache's coming back.

ME: Sniff another apple.

BEN: Yes dear.

ME: For the yellow sun design on the roof of the hut and maybe the banisters, this yellow felt-tip pen is about right. And there's a yellow dress I like on Kate Winslet in Celebrity Weekly – look.

BEN: Very nice (sniffing apple), I'll have a search on the internet.

BEN: I've found some paint colours I think you'll like – your turn to look now. The yellow was trickier to find in exterior ranges. Most are sandy coloured.

ME: Maybe I could use a sandy shade on the flooring.... This is a nice yellow (scrolling).

BEN: It's called dazzling yellow.

ME: I like it. Looks like daffodil yellow (more scrolling) and this blue is beautiful, I'll call it beach hut blue..... this one is really nice too, I'll call it seaside blue.

BEN: This one (scrolling) we'll call Herne Bay blue (laughing).

ME: Yes!

BEN: I'll order you a paint chart to peruse (crunching an apple).

ME: Thanks (sniffing an apple).

Monday 2nd

11.27 a.m. I'm engrossed in a posh-looking paint chart from Farrow & Ball – the eco-friendly paint people.

ME: There's some delicately beautiful shades and radiant shades that are gorgeous, with interesting names – some strange, some comical, many intriguing. Sulking room pink..... Stiffkey blue...... Calluna..... Cromarty.... Wevet.

BEN: There's explanations for each colour on the back of the chart.

ME: Oh goody....... Sulking room pink is a muted, rose colour evocative of the colours used in boudoirs, a room originally named after the French word bouder – to sulk...... Stiffkey blue is an inky blue named after the North Norfolk beach where the mud, along with the cockles, has a particular blue hue. If I had a beach hut on the Norfolk coast I would paint it that colour, along with grey shades to match the lovely wild seals we saw there once (eyes far away in Norfolk).

BEN: What about Calluna, Cromarty and Wevet?

ME: Erm......... here we are. Calluna is a tranquil lilac that takes its name from the beautiful heather, so prolific across the moors in Scotland........ The muted green-grey, Cromarty, is named after the Firth estuary, a place of swirling mists, mentioned daily in the shipping forecast..... I like Mizzle. It's a soft green-grey, named after West Country evening skies, when there's a mix of both mist and drizzle. I've seen this on camping holidays (eyes far away in the West Country).

BEN: You've drifted away again. Come home dear. What's Wevet?

ME: Just a mo.... Here it is. It's such a delicate white with a translucent, gossamer feel, it's named after the old Dorset term for spider's web (eyes far away on the coast of Dorset).

BEN: Come home from Dorset!.......... I like the Cooking Apple green (biting into a Braeburn).

ME: There should be colours named after apples, like Golden Delicious and Granny Smith.

BEN: Yeah (crunch, munch).

ME: I like like the sound of this colour – Borrowed Light. Evoking the colour of summer skies, it's named after the delicate light that cascades through small windows...... I must find it on the chart....... here it is...... it's the palest, duck egg blue. Lovely.

BEN: What are you like (munch, crunch).

ME: If I had the energy, I'd like to paint the hut stripes, the colours of the pebbles on the beach. There are so many soft, creamy, grey, grey-blue and toffee shades. As well as the Wevet white.... Ammonite... Stony ground.... Calamine.... Worsted.... String.

BEN: Would you like Bill and I to paint those colours for you?

ME: Oh no! Wouldn't want to put you to *that much* effort. And anyway, all the different paints would be bloomim' expensive. A lovely blue will be perfect. I like Cook's Blue, inspired by the rich, romantic finish found in the cook's closet at Calke Abbey. But I think my favourite one is St Giles Blue, a vivid and striking blue, inspired by the hall at St Giles House in the quaint area of Wimborne, St Giles.

BEN: When I'm in town, I'll see what I can find in Wilko.

2.32 p.m.   Ben returns home from town with pain killers, apples, a big, fresh loaf and two small pots of paint.

BEN: I popped into Homebase and Wilko. Here you are. Two little tester pots.

ME: Ooh, the St Giles blue looks lovely. The brilliant yellow is delightfully bright – will make a perfect sunshine design against the beautiful blue. I'll find a piece of old wood in the cellar and paint a little blue hut with sunshine design on the roof, right away. I do hope I get my hut!

BEN: Fingers crossed.

ME: Broomsticks crossed.

BEN: How's the witchy book you're writing going?

ME: Very well..... But it's not just a follow-up to my first witchy book, it's a sort of follow-up to a diary style book I wrote too. Don't know if it'll work but I'm having a go. I've had a break from writing the first draft in pencil, wasn't sure about it. Think I'll start the rewrite tomorrow in pencil. I could type it on my lovely new laptop in my beach hut. I will be like the late writer, Roald Dahl.

BEN: Did he write his books in a beach hut?

ME: He wrote in a shed at the bottom of his garden. I think a hut at the top of the beach will be more fun – the sea air refreshing the brain cells.

BEN: Yeah.

ME: I have something in common with Roald. He liked to eat chocolate when he wrote. I expect it oiled his creative cogs. He rolled – or should I say Roald – empty chocolate wrappers into a ball, that eventually became about tennis ball size. It still sits on his desk next to the old chair he used to sit in to write. Judging by the purple colour of the choc wrapper ball, I think he liked Cadbury's milk chocolate. Plain gets my brain working better.

BEN: I'm nipping back into town to get guitar strings and a bar of plain choc.

ME: Lovely (licking lips). How's the composing going?

BEN: Really good. Nine tracks almost finished. One more to go.

ME: I expect cheese and beer helps the old brain cogs.

BEN: It does. When all the tunes are finished, I'll put them on a CD so you can have a listen, and help me decide on the titles.

ME: It will be my pleasure!

Tuesday 3rd

ME: It's very chilly and overcast today. I hope it's sunny when you and Bill go to Herne Bay to look at the hut.

BEN: Yeah.

ME: Best wrap up well if it's like today – it'll be chillier at the coast. You forgot your cap last time.

BEN: Certainly dear.

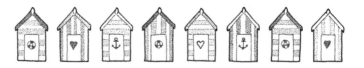

1.33 p.m.   I decide to get down to my witchy/diary rewrite, ready to type beside the seaside, beside the sea. I sing a little song as I switch the kettle on, open a bar of smooth, mellow, dark chocolate, and snap off a piece.

Oh! I do like to be beside the seaside
Oh! I will like to type beside the sea
And I will love to tap the little keys, keys, keys
As I breathe in a very beautiful sea, sea, breeze

1.38 p.m.   I start scribbling away with a nice, sharp, red 2B pencil. On a nice, shiny, black, new A4 spiral note-pad. A nice, clean, white pencil eraser at the ready. The grey writing cogs in my brain, are shiny and nicely oiled with smooth, dark brown chocolate.

MARCH

Monday 1st

8.46 a.m.

ME: *I've been offered a place at leap-frog college.*

BEN: *Are you sure dear?*

ME: *Oh yes. I jumped at the chance (cackling).*

BEN: *Ah (smiling), is it a leap year?*

ME: *It may be! I think my broomstick is going to need a jump-start before I ride it again. It's been so long since I last rode it, because of the lockdown.*

BEN: *Don't you mean a bump-start? A jump-start is when you use jump leads.*

ME: *To get my broomstick going I need you, once I'm off* the ground a bit, to push me from behind and jump up and down making frog noises. Remember?

BEN: Oh yes. I expect the neighbours remember too.

ME: And I sing Paul McCartney's Frog Song.

> **Win or lose, sink or swim**
> **One thing is certain we'll never give in**
> **Side by side, hand in hand**
> **We'll all stand together**

BEN: I imagine the neighbours remember that too. I think you've forgotten I got you a brand new, super-speed broomstick for your birthday. You have such a leaky cauldron brain.

ME: Oh yes (eyes lighting up like a candle).

10.05 a.m.

ME: I've got it!

BEN: The joke I told you yesterday?

ME: I got that (smiling).

BEN: How to work the DVD player?

ME: I'll never get that..... I got the answer to a riddle I heard on the radio.

BEN: *Do you feel like a clever witch?*

ME: *I do. The radio presenter gave us half an hour to come up with the answer, and I got it in under a minute! I texted the answer to the station and it was lovely to hear my name on the radio. I felt famous for –*

BEN: *Two seconds?*

ME: *Yes (quietly cackling).*

BEN: *What was the riddle and the answer?*

ME: *I'll tell you the riddle but let you guess the answer.*

Always old
Sometimes new

BEN: *I'm no good at riddles.... My socks?*

ME: *There's more.*

Never sad
Sometimes blue

BEN: *Haven't, haven't got a clue.*

ME: **Never empty
Sometimes full**

BEN: *My stomach?*

ME: **Never pushy
Sometimes pull**

BEN: *The barmaid at The Pilot?*

ME: *Do you need a clue?*

BEN: *Yeah.*

ME: *When it's full it's a perfect time for witches to fly on their broomsticks.*

BEN: *A goblet full of golden mead at Summer Solstice?*

ME: *No, but this is your final clue. Some old witches only fly once in a blue -*

BEN: *Got it!*

ME: *You got it after the first clue didn't you.*

BEN: *Yep.*

6.30 p.m. I'm watching *Holidaying with Jane McDonald: Florida*. The singer is on a road trip through the American state, beginning by picking up her car in

Orlando and heading off for a self-kayaking excursion.

ME: Jane McDonald is having a great time self-kayaking in Florida on Channel 5. Looks *so much fun!*

BEN: Don't go getting any ideas dear, now that you could soon be the owner of a second-hand kayak.

WE LAUGH

Wednesday 4th

9.06 a.m.

BEN: Chilly again (turning the heating up).

ME: Yes. So rainy, dull and cloudy, it feels like the end instead of the beginning of summer. People are plodding past the house wearing wintry weather clothing – dark blues and green back-to-school September colours. What will the weather do? It could be the coldest, wettest summer on record. And if I get the hut it could be too wet and cold for you to renovate it. And the man selling the hut may change his mind anyway, wanting one of his children to inherit it. And the man on Radio Kent this morning said hail and thunder is expected. The cost of living is going up as the number of Covid infections come down. And the news about war gets worse. And I'm starting a headache.

BEN: Sniff an apple dear (handing me a Braeburn).

ME: Thanks. I'll get back to writing my witchy diary. That'll cheer me up.

9.26 a.m.   I continue with the second half of *Monday 1st March* – I'll be smiling in no time.

ME: *I'll be so happy to be out riding on my broomstick again when yet another lockdown is over.*

BEN: *The film Destry Rides Again is on this afternoon. You will be Verity Rides Again.*

ME: *That could be the title of my next book.*

BEN: *Yeah.*

ME: *It's been almost a year since I met with my witchy sisters. Witches are good at social distancing and wearing masks when restrictions are lifted. But I have friends who have to attend the very sick. They do their caring work on the frontline of the NHS – though on-one knows in private, they are good, healing witches. Some of them have caught the virus and taken quite a while to recover, so it's probably best I don't meet up with them for now.*

BEN: *When witches are in their bubble with family, are they in a hubble bubble?*

ME: *Of course (quietly cackling). And I'm so looking forward to my next merry meet with my sisters.*

We merry meet

> *With merry mead*
> *Wearing black*
> *And yellow tweed*

BEN: **And cook with**
Coriander seed

ME: *You make me cackle! I miss the bats from the bottom of the garden joining me for a flight. Then an owl and a little dragon appearing, hooting and squealing around my pointy hat. Though I do feel we'll be social distancing and wearing masks for many moons to come.*

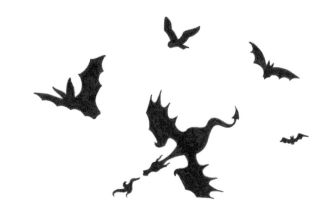

BEN: *Yeah.*

ME: *When it's full moon I feel restless and want to go out flying, but I've been doing some spell work to take my mind off how I'm feeling and full moon is a good time for healing spells. I've done them for my family, your family and sister witches to help them recover from the Covid.*

BEN: *I'm sure they'll benefit (smiling).*

ME: *My penfriend Jim sent me a photo of a very pretty red wax-cap fungi on a lawn. I must send a copy of it to my niece, she loves toadstools and mushrooms in fairytale illustrations. Can you print me out a copy please?*

BEN: *No problem.*

ME: *Lovely. I miss my little witch, Louise.*

BEN: *Not so little anymore, she towers over you.*

ME: *I can't believe she's in her twenties now. But she will always be my little witch.*

BEN: *That doesn't surprise me.*

ME: I'm looking forward to when I can fly over to see her again on my super-speed broomstick. It will take half the time it used to, to get to her town.

BEN: No need for a frog jump-start.

ME: Yes! And Louise loves the new broomstick we gave her for Christmas. My sister used it to sweep her yard and got it very grubby because she'd had some building work done. Louise was very unhappy about this and decided to leave the broomstick outside overnight so the rain would clean it.

BEN: Did the storm with all the lightning energize it?

ME: I'm sure it did. Louise said it looked good as new the next day and sort of glowed. Her cat, Felicity, likes to use it as a scratching post now. She sent a sweet text message – look.

HI AUNTIE, MY CAT LIKES TO SCRATCH MY BROOMSTICK – I THINK SHE IS MAKING FRIENDS WITH IT AND PUTTING HER SCENT ON IT WITH HER MUZZLE, AND SHE WOULD LIKE TO FLY ON MY BROOMSTICK WITH ME WHEN I GO OUT AFTER LOCKDOWN

I replied:

I THINK MY CATS WANT TO FLY WITH ME ON MY BROOMSTICK TOO – THEY HAVE BEEN DOING THE SAME THING – I MUST

LOOZ SOME LOCKDOWN WEIGHT SO I DON'T ADD EXTRA
WEIGHT TO THE BROOM, AS WELL AS HAVING TWO WELL
FED CATS RIDING BEHIND ME MAKING IT GO SLOWER

Louise replied:

ME TOO – CACKLE, CACKLE XXX

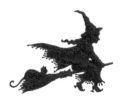

Thursday 5th

8.23 a.m.

ME: I dreamt last night that you and I were in kayaks, madly rowing towards a beach to be in time for something. I can't remember what.

BEN: Did we get there in time?

ME: We did! It may be my witchy senses telling me that all will be fine with the beach hut.

BEN: I'm sure you're right dear.

8.25 a.m. I gaze up into the pale blue, early summer sky, as I spread peanuts on the bird table. I think my Farrow & Ball paint chart would describe the sky as Lulworth blue – the shade of the sea at the beautiful Lulworth Cove in Dorset. Maybe that's the shade of blue I should paint my hut.

It's cold today. The breeze whipping my hair across my

eyes. I brush it away and smile at sunshine sparkling on the rain-soaked garden. I love the glowing greens. I touch the leaves on the hedge, raindrops trickling down my fingers. The Farrow & Ball chart would say it's Calke green – a rich, dark green found in the breakfast room in Calke Abbey. Maybe the decking on my beach hut could be this colour.

The bluebells nod their delicate heads in the breeze, I think they are agreeing with me. I love their shade of blue, reminding me of the colour I'm thinking of painting my hut. I think I will stay with the colour I have chosen, it looked good when I painted a little hut with the tester pot on a piece of wood.

I love the greens and blues in the garden
Rain soaked deep into their roots
While pixies dance at the end of the lawn
In their little pixie boots

8.30 a.m. I evenly spread honey on wholemeal toast and think of my beach hut. It has endured many, many years of chilling winds from the North Sea. Baking, cheese bubbling pizza hut – I mean pizza hot, sun. Freezing, gale force something gales. Endless rainfall and heavy Herne Bay hail stones. It will so enjoy a fresh coat of beautiful blue paint, spread evenly and lovingly over its weary weathered woodwork after a good clean and undercoat.

I can see myself cosy in my hut writing poetry in all weathers.

I watch heavy Herne Bay hail
And a ship without a sail

I admire a seagull soaring
And my nice new beach hut flooring
Enjoy a mug of minty tea
And the swimmers in the sea

The sound of children's laughter
It's my happy ever after

8.31 a.m.   I crunch honey on toast, my thoughts still with my hut in Herne Bay.

You've endured freezing gales
Fresh from the coast
You'll enjoy a nice new coat
Like honey spread on toast

9.35 a.m.   I'm in the mood to continue with my witchy diary (still in the month of March) while my brain is still creatively fresh – the cogs oiled with golden honey.

Tuesday 2nd

ME: *It's World Wildlife Day.*

BEN: *Well, we're certainly doing our bit (lugging a huge sack of peanuts into the kitchen).*

ME: *We are. Our squirrels and birdies look very well fed.*

BEN: *The fox family and hedgehogs too.*

ME: *And me and you.*

BEN: *True..... I hear some verse coming on.*

ME: *Birds and squirrels are well fed*
Foxes, hedgehogs too

BEN: *And I will have to add to that*
The cats and me and you

WE LAUGH

11.06 a.m.

ME: *Louise is mad about hedgehogs. She has a tattoo of one on her arm. She likes foxes and squirrels as well as owls now.*

BEN: *I wonder where she gets it from (laughing).*

ME: *I'm wondering how she's coping with the lockdown. Think I'll text her.*

HI LOUISE, HOW ARE YOU COPING WITH ANOTHER LOCKDOWN LITTLE WITCH ?

11.22 a.m.

ME: *You sound very happy. Heard you whistling away merrily in the kitchen.*

BEN: *I am. My music is going really well. I'm writing a brilliant piano solo – though I say it myself.*

ME: *Great! The bass line and guitar is sounding very*

lovely and the drums are really groovy.

BEN: *Thanks.*

ME: *It'll be so good when the restaurant you played at before the pandemic employs you again.*

BEN: *Yeah.*

ME: *I heard a song on the radio earlier by Frank Sinatra that could be another one for your set. The older generation in your audience will remember it.*

       When I was seventeen
       It was a very good year
       It was a very good year
       For small town girls

BEN: *I'll get my guitar.*

ME: *I've written my own version of a verse of the song.*

BEN: *Am I surprised? (smiling).*

ME: *In twenty twenty-one*
       It wasn't a very good year

> *It wasn't a very good year*
> *For musician boys*

BEN: *You're right there (picking up guitar and working out chords to the song)...... Em....... F....... Em...... G....... F...... E...... D.....*

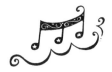

11.52 a.m.   *Louise replied to my text message:*

HI AUNTIE, I-M OK – I MISS MY MATES AND HAVING MY LONG WITCHY NAILS DONE BUT I'VE BEEN COOKING – CAN YOU SEND ME SOME WITCHY RECIPES FOR BAKING A CAKE ?

I replied:

OF COURSE – WILL PERUSE MY WITCHY COOKBOOK XX

11.55 a.m.   *Louise replies:*

COOL – THANX AUNTIE XX

Friday 6th

10.00 a.m.

ME: *Another day*
       Chilly and wet
       I think that Lovely

Needs the vet

One glance at the calendar
No, not yet

BEN: *My music needs a mix*
           My car needs a fix

           Our next door neighbour
           Is up to his old tricks

ME: *Two birds are on*
           The bird table fighting

           Time for me to
           Knuckle down to writing

10.23 a.m. I continue with March.

Wednesday 3rd

8.46 a.m.

BEN: *Coffee?*

ME: *Yes. Your real coffee please.*

BEN: *Gone off the decaf?*

ME: *No, I just fancy a bit of a lift.*

BEN: *A broomstick riding lift?*

ME: *More a mental lift. And a bit of a buzz.*

BEN: *Buzzy bee honey on toast too? I got a jar of Rob's honey from his hives when I saw him yesterday.*

ME: *Made by very happy bees.*

BEN: *How do you know they are very happy?*

ME: *Because Rob has happy hens, or his girls, as he calls them, that he looks after well. So I imagine he looks after his bees too. They need a lot of care. The hive needs to be kept –*

BEN: *Bee-kept.*

ME: *Yes dear. It needs to be kept dry, airy and clean. And the colony checked regularly to make sure they are doing well, and extra frames added in peak season. I wonder if vets come out to see bees if they seem unwell. You can't really take a hive along to the vets can you. Imagine sitting in a waiting room with a little hive on your lap, bees buzzing round your head.*

BEN: *Only you could imagine that dear.*

WE LAUGH

ME: *Their hum has to be just right. If they are noisy their food supply is low. But you can give them sugar syrup towards the end of the summer.*

BEN: *They like to hum when they don't know the words to a song.*

ME: *Yes (quietly cackling). Or maybe they need a coffee.*

BEN: *Coffee?*

ME: *Bees enjoy a coffee boost like us. Caffeine can be found in the nectar of many plants, like citrus blossoms, not just the coffee plant. Bees seem to prefer caffeinated nectar!*

BEN: *I wonder if Rob brings his bees a morning coffee.*

ME: *Coffee with sugar at the end of the summer.*

BEN: *I can see you writing a book about happy bees who meet for a coffee and a chat.*

ME: *I'd write it for my little niece who loves honey.*

9.16 a.m.

BEN: *I see you're scribbling away. Has the coffee and honey given you the buzz you need?*

ME: *Definitely. I'm writing notes for a book for Louise entitled, Bee Happy.*

9.16 p.m.   I'm watching *Agatha Christie's Marple*. A distraught, posh lady has just said, worse things happen at sea. I hope good things will happen by the sea for me soon.

Worse things happen at sea
Worse things happen at sea
I hope that something nice will happen
Beach hut wise to me

Broomsticks crossed.

Saturday 7th

9.27 a.m.

ME: I dreamt we were kayaking again last night.

BEN: That's nice (yawning).

ME: It wasn't nice. We were rowing along, being chased by a monster shark. I wondered why I dreamt this until I noticed in TV Weekly just now, a photo taken from above, of two people rowing kayaks followed by a shark, three times the size of their kayaks. It was advertising the film, *The Reef: Stalked*. Two women, Annie and Nik, embark on a kayaking trip with their female friends and find themselves menaced by a great white shark.

BEN: Did we escape from the shark in your dream?

ME: Yes.

BEN: Phew (wiping brow).

ME: This could mean we will overcome obstacles in the future.

BEN: I'm sure you're right dear.

9.41 a.m.   It's a cloudy day. I used to enjoy a nice, relaxing bit of cloud watching..... a hippo with wings..... chasing a dragon with long legs..... a hedgehog about to eat a cupcake. But this is not possible anymore, unless I plod into the garden, since the new housing estate was built opposite our house. BUT when I get my beach hut I will be able to sit in comfort with a cuppa, watching clouds sailing across the sky over the sea to my heart's content....... a fat dolphin...... chases a seahorse with teeth........ about to eat a currant bun........ that morphs into a rowing boat.

9.42 a.m.   On Radio Kent, Erica North is chatting to a weather girl. She tells the girl that her radio station is based in Herne Bay, and when there's a forecast in our part of the country, the weather is often a little better in Herne Bay. The weather girl says you do get places like that. Gravesend is one of them. This is good to know.

10.00 a.m. I'm in the mood to get back to more rewriting of witchy diary now. Still in the month of March.

Thursday 4th

ME: Do you know what day it is?

BEN: Thursday? Recycling day? De-flea a cat day? Tesco delivery day? World Wide Witches' Day?

ME: It is Thursday. A delivery day. A cat de-flea day. But it's also World Book Day. People have been calling into Radio Kent to say what book they are reading at the moment.

BEN: Thrilling.

ME: What are you reading at the moment?

BEN: The Indian takeaway and pizza delivery flyers that have just come with the post.

ME: Very funny.

BEN: Actually I'm reading, How to live a peaceful life with your partner during a lockdown.

ME: Who is the author?

BEN: Miss Havina Nicelife (laughing).

ME: Lucky her, havin' a nice name. Do you know what else is nice?

BEN: *Can't wait to hear.*

ME: *Children are being encouraged to read books and dress up as their favourite character in a book they like – then do a zoom call with friends.*

BEN: *When you are next zooming off to a merry-meet on your super-speed broomstick, and you call me on your mobile on the way, will that be a zoom call?*

ME: *Witches NEVER use their mobile phone when they are riding on a broomstick. It's easy to lose concentration when you are blethering and cackling away, and end up crashing into a tree or a chimney pot.*

BEN: *Or TV ariel. I should have realised (laughing).*

ME: *When witches do zoom calls to sister witches, guess what they call them?*

BEN: *Can't imagine.*

ME: *Besom calls. Bee-zoom calls.*

BEN: *That must give them a buzz!*

6.30 p.m.   *I send a text message to my niece:*

HI LITTLE WITCH, WHAT WAS YOUR FAVE BOOK WHEN YOU
WERE A VERY LITTLE WITCH ?

6.36 p.m.   *Louise replied:*

HI AUNTIE, MY FAVE BOOK WHEN I WAS LITTLE WAS THE
ONE YOU WROTE - LOVE AND BEST WITCHES. THE WORST
WITCH WAS A GOOD BOOK TOO - WHAT WAS YOUR FAVE
BOOK ?

6.37 p.m.   *I replied:*

I LOVED THE LION THE WITCH AND THE WARDROBE - AND
ALL THE NARNIA BOOKS - THANK YOU FOR LIKING MY BOOK
BEST - YOU HAVE MADE AN OLD WITCH VERY HAPPY XXX

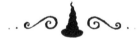

9.16 p.m.   I'm watching *Lighthouses: Building The Impossible*.
Rob Bell explores the bizarre history of The Smalls,
one of Britain's most remote offshore lighthouses,
situated twenty miles off the Pembrokeshire coast.

ME: I remember seeing some lighthouse ornaments I
liked, years ago when we were in Dungeness. I think
a little lighthouse would look good in my beach hut. I
want to give it a homely feel with a few ornaments
on a shelf.

BEN: Doesn't surprise me.

ME: I take it you haven't heard from the Beach Hut Association man, Andrew yet.

BEN: Nope.

Sunday 8th

11.00 a.m.   It's a beautiful day. The sun shines brightly, reminding us that summer is on its way. There's a buzzing sound of neighbours mowing their lawns, and I open the kitchen window, letting the grassy fragrance flow in.

ME: I like the smell of fresh mown grass. One of the smells of summer. Don't you?

BEN: Yeah. I like the of smell toast and coffee too.

ME: Fancy a coffee?

BEN: Please.

ME: Toast?

BEN: Yeah.

ME: Do you know, the poet William Wordsworth who –

BEN: Wandered lonely as a cloud?

ME: Yes. He didn't have a sense of smell! How sad that he wrote about the beauty of daffodils but didn't experience their wonderful springtime fragrance. How different his Wordsworth words would have been. He loved to grow wildflowers at his home, in his garden at Dove Cottage in the Lake District, and like me, loved daisies. He wrote about them.

BEN: You wrote about daisies once didn't you?

ME: I recall writing about feeling as fresh as a daisy under a cow pat!

BEN: Having no sense of smell would have been useful to Wordsworth when he wandered lonely as a cloud among the cow pats.

ME: *He wandered lonely as a cow pat*
Among the cows that go moo
Then came home tired at sunset
Something smelly on his shoe

WE LAUGH

ME: I was reading; when you smell coffee, you're breathing in around four hundred different molecules, of which about a third contribute to the odour – it's a kind of chord of smell. You often find the same molecules reoccurring in unexpected places. There's a molecule in coffee that you also find in the smell of fresh bread and cucumber.

BEN: Fascinating. I'm off to Sainsbury's for some beers later, want anything?

ME: Mmm..... A loaf of fresh bread would be nice and a cucumber for a salad sandwich. We've got toms and lettuce. I fancy a salad for dinner, how about you?

BEN: Yeah.

ME: Okay. Get a nice quiche and some coleslaw. We've got peppers.

BEN: Shall I get potato salad, Sains do a nice one – save making it.

ME: Sounds good. I'll make a list.

BEN: Okay.

ME: Look at these black tomatoes in Weekly Witch.

BEN: Are you sure they're tomatoes?

ME: Yes. They are a new breed of tomato. Supposed to be healthier than their red cousins. The indigo rose species was cultivated by scientists in America, who bred regular red tomatoes with wild varieties that contain anthocyanin – an antioxidant that may help obesity and diabetes. Starting life as a regular - looking green tomato, it gradually ripens to a dramatic jet black.

BEN: Very witchy.

ME: With purple carrots and green cauliflower available, we could have some very witchy looking meals!

BEN: Yes dear.

ME: I must get down to more rewriting of my witchy diary before my old brain dozes off.

BEN: How's it going?

ME: Well, thanks. *Friday the fifth of March* today. Not much deleting or rewriting, mostly recipes.

BEN: Good. Right I'm off.

ME: Hang on, I'll just write your list.

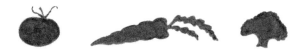

Friday 5th

1.06 p.m.   I leaf through my old, weary, weathered Real
            Witches' Kitchen cookbook, searching for a recipe
            or two, to send to my niece. Then I write her a
            letter on my best witchy writing paper.

            Dear Louise

            Here's a recipe I think you'll like, for a simple
            sponge cake, with ideas for added ingredients.

            4oz butter
            4oz caster sugar
            2 beaten eggs
            4oz self raising flour

            Cream the butter and sugar together, beat in the
            eggs and stir in the flour. Turn into a greased and
            floured eight inch tin (better than turning into a
            frog!). Bake at 180° C/ 350° F for 25 to 30 minutes.
            Test with a skewer to see whether it's done (if the
            skewer comes out clean the cake is cooked).

My witchy cookbook says this recipe can form a basis for any number of variations. I thought you'd like to add cocoa powder and chocolate chips or ground coconut and white chocolate buttons. The book doesn't mention the weight of added ingredients but I'm sure your mum will guide you.

Love & Best Witches Auntie xxx

P.S.   *After I finished your letter I came across a recipe for a cake that is eaten by witches on 21st March (the Spring Equinox when day and night are equal). It's the festival of Oestara. Simnel cake is baked this time of year. It's just a basic sponge cake mix with nutmeg, cinnamon, ginger and mixed spice. Two cakes are baked, sandwiched together with marzipan and decorated with marzipan eggs.*

If you'd like to make your own marzipan, here are the ingredients:

½ pound icing sugar
½ pound caster sugar
1 pound ground almonds
1 teaspoon vanilla essence or extract
2 eggs

Lemon juice

Sift the icing sugar into a bowl and add the sugar and ground almonds. Add the vanilla essence. Lightly beat the eggs and add, together with enough lemon juice to make a stiff dough. Knead lightly and roll out. Try not to let the paste dry out, as it will crack – like my leaky old cauldron!

HAPPY BAKING X

1.16 p.m.   *I notice a recipe for a soup eaten at the festival of Oestara. Nettle soup. I write it down as a reminder for myself because we have lots of nettles in the garden about to be cut down and I'd like to make the soup. Although we must leave some growing for the butterflies to enjoy.*

1 lb nettle leaves

2 cloves of freshly chopped garlic
1oz butter
1/2 pint vegetable stock
1 pint whole milk

Wash and chop the nettle leaves and fry with the garlic in butter. Add the stock, bring to the boil and simmer for five minutes. Blend through a sieve. Add the milk and heat gently. Serve with a swirl of cream and fresh bread.

Sounds delicious. I'm sure Ben will be as thrilled as when I suggested nettle tea to help his hay fever.

1.26 p.m.   *I sent Louise a text:*

HI LOUISE, AS WELL AS CAKE RECIPES WOULD YOU LIKE
TO MAKE NETTLE SOUP, IF YOUR MUM HAS NETTLES
GROWING IN HER GARDEN ?

1.30 p.m.   *Louise replied:*

YES PLZ – THAT WOULD BE WITCHY FUN – WE'VE GOT LOTS
OF NETTLES AT THE END OF OUR GARDEN X

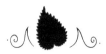

7.12 p.m.   I'm watching *Villages By The Sea* and thinking of a little beach hut village by the sea.

ME: Have you heard from Andrew, the beach hut association man yet?

BEN: No dear.

Monday 9th

8.06 a.m. The early morning sun blazes through a gap in the bedroom curtains. Golden fingers of light gently stroke Diamanda's silky, black head. I softly sing to her as I caress her warm coat. She purrs. A beautiful contented, silky, black purr.

The sun has got his hat on
Hip, hip, hip hurray!
The sun has got his hat on
And he's coming out to play

ME: I've got a good feeling about today.

BEN: Oh good (yawning).

8.26 a.m. The kettle is boiling. Toast is toasting. Eggs with golden yolks from happy hens are bubbling away. Lovely pads silently into the kitchen through the cat flap on her huge, grey, fluffy paws. I stroke her soft, grey head, give her a little scratch behind the ears and under the chin. She purrs. A prize winning purr.

ME: Herne Bay got a mention on Radio Kent again earlier.

BEN: Yeah?

ME: There was a chap talking about the recovery of the retail industry from the pandemic lockdowns. Many people, like us, are shopping online now. He was asked which places in the high street were doing best. The first town he mentioned was Herne Bay. Then Whitstable and Margate. Maybe people feel safer from the virus in places by the sea, with fresh sea breezes. I was thinking, we could advertise the kayak in Herne Bay high street.

BEN: Yeah.

10.36 a.m.   Time for another cuppa and more rewriting of witchy diary, still in the month of March.

Sunday 6th

6.30 p.m.   *Louise sends me a text:*

> HI AUNTIE, MUM IS TEACHING ME HOW TO BAKE BREAD – I'M GOING TO MAKE BREAD ROLLS – MUM SAYS THEY ARE NICE WITH HOME-MADE SOUP – CAN YOU SEND ME ANOTHER RECIPE FOR SOUP AS WELL AS THE NETTLE SOUP ?

6.32 p.m.   *I have a feeling Louise has gone off the idea, or my sister is not keen on the idea of nettle soup, as I reply:*

> OF COURSE, IT WILL BE A PLEASURE – WILL SEND SOON WITH SOME HERBS I HAVE GROWN IN MY GARDEN X

Louise replied:

> THAT WILL BE COOL – THANX AUNTIE X

6.40 p.m.   *As I turn to **S** in the index of The Real Witches' Kitchen to find soups, I recall that Louise likes sweetcorn and a thick, hearty soup. So I find a pad and pencil and get scribbling.*

Sweetcorn Chowder

2 potatoes
1 onion
1 tin drained sweetcorn
1 tin tomatoes
2 pints water
1 tbsp cornflower
½ pint milk

Peel and dice the potatoes and onion. Place them, together with the sweetcorn and tomatoes, in water, bring to the boil and simmer for 15 minutes. Add the cornflower and milk, blend well and add to the soup. Warm through until the cornflower has thickened and serve.

6.42 p.m.   *I make a note to put sweetcorn, cornflower and potatoes on tomorrow's shopping delivery list, and see if I can order a new cauldron on the internet.*

11.04 a.m.

BEN: I've just got a text from Andrew (frowning).

ME: Oh dear. Has the beach hut owner changed his mind

and decided not to sell? Has the hut burned down? Has it fallen apart and blown away in gale force something winds?

BEN: All's fine. Just wanted to see your face (smiling).

ME: Oh, good (sigh of relief). Has Andrew got the keys for the hut now?

BEN: Yep. And he'll arrange a date for the viewing.

ME: Hurrah!

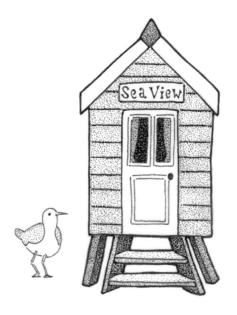

Chapter Two

May

Tuesday 10th

9.46 a.m.

BEN: I'm meeting Andrew at five o'clock this afternoon at the hut, with Bill.

ME: Great! The weather girl said there will be plenty of sunshine heading your way.

Zip-a-dee-doo-dah, Zip-a-dee-ay
My, oh, my, what a wonderful day

BEN: *Plenty of sunshine headin' my way*

ME: *Zip-a-dee-doo-dah, zip-a-dee-ay*

WE LAUGH

BEN: Bill is all set to go. He suggested we take a torch so we can look up under the eaves in the hut.

ME: Good thinking.

BEN: I'll charge-up our torch so it's at it's brightest.

ME: Brilliant. I'll keep my broomsticks crossed that the hut isn't in a bad condition inside. And things that need doing are do-able.

10.07 a.m.

BEN: How's the book going?

ME: Good. But I'm feeling too excited and a little app-
       rehensive to get down to rewriting today. I'll just
       read a few pages to decide how much I'd like to
       delete or keep.

10.09 a.m.   Perusing my witchy diary, I think I'll delete the bits
              about the pandemic on the news, Ben getting ill from
              a Covid jab, me deciding not to have the jab after
              reading about the effect it can have on people with
              ME, and the mention of our bereavements. My witchy
              and happy storylines are much more fun.

10.29 a.m.   I watch *A Place In The Sun*. A couple, Ashley and
              Justin, are looking for a place to live beside the sea-
              side in Spain, with a beautiful sea view.

10.34 a.m.   I enjoy a beautiful beach-hut-beside-the-seaside-in-
              Herne Bay daydream, and don't feel the *slightest bit*
              envious of Ashley and Justin.

1.00 p.m.   Engrossed in Weekly Wife, I'm interested to read that
              natural light increases levels of the happy hormone
              serotonin, which boosts energy and mood. I'll be
              full of happy hormones at my beach hut, with lots
              of natural light beside the seaside, and find energy to
              plod on the pebbles.

1.21 p.m.   As I nibble a digestive biscuit with a minty cuppa, I
              imagine keeping a biscuit tin in my hut. I've got a
              beautiful biscuit barrel with a decorative, colo-
              urful, fruit design – a Christmas gift full of fruity
              biscuits. It was soon empty. I could go mad and fill it
              with two varieties of biscuits *and* KitKats.

              When the hut is clean and decorated and I 'move
              in', I'll bring a box of supplies. Teas, coffee, bottled

water. Kitchen roll, loo roll, matches. Cans of soup with a ring-pull, to heat up on chilly days. On hot days I could bring Tupperware boxes full of tasty salad things for lunch. Ben and I could sit outside the hut, looking very chic on the powder blue bistro set advertised in Weekly Wife, echoing the clean tones of harbour homes – folding steel to fit neatly in the corner of the hut when we go home. Although on second thoughts, our soft canvas chairs will be more comfortable.

2.30 p.m.   I almost cut my finger, slicing cucumber for a salad sandwich, and decide a little first aid kit in the hut may be a good idea.

2.32 p.m.   My hands feel dry. I'll keep a small tube of hand cream in the first aid box. And a lip salve.

2.34 p.m.   As I pile some clothes into the washing machine, I decide to keep a warm jumper at the hut, in case I'm there on a day when it suddenly turns chillier than expected.

2.36 p.m.   Sitting in the garden with Diamanda and Lovely, I enjoy my sandwich, al fresco. Then leaf through a gift catalogue, fluttering through the pages like the white butterfly nearby, fluttering over the nettles, until my eyes alight on the seaside section.

2.38 p.m.   I almost squawk like a seagull, with delight when I spot the deckchair with a bright, puffins design – black, white and blue with their lovely red and yellow striped beaks, on a blue background – the same blue as my hut is going to be.

2.39 p.m.   The beach front bather ornament, a lady wearing a blue and white striped swimming costume, holding a red and white beach ball, is amusing. So is her friend, wearing a pink and blue striped costume, holding a red and white lifebelt. Both ladies are rather large – recalling vintage seaside postcards. Maybe I should order one of them to sit next to the biscuit tin, as a reminder not to overindulge.

2.46 p.m.   I sneeze and take a tissue out of my cardie pocket. I'll keep tissues and maybe some Lemsip at the hut.

3.15 p.m.   Time for another cuppa (and maybe not another biscuit) and a peruse of Celebrity Weekly. There's a double-page spread of an **A** to **Z** of things that can make you happy. The two I like best are **B** & **S**.

B is for blue space. Studies have found being near water – blue space – whether it's on a beach or by a lake, pond or river, floods our brains with feel-good hormones and drains away stress too. So find a stretch of water to walk by or simply sit and soak up the atmosphere.

Sitting in my beach hut, eating al fresco, will be simply *parfait*.

S is for search for a natural, pretty object. Take a stroll somewhere you love and find a seashell or a pebble. You should be able to recapture a feeling of calm whenever you look at it.

I will sit on the edge of the decking of my hut and pick up a pebble, then take it home and place it on the side of the bath. And when I'm enjoying a bubble bath, I will bubble-up with happy seaside thoughts. And maybe sing a little song about how I do like to be beside the seaside.

3.36 p.m.   In Weekly Wife there is also an **A** to **Z**. This time it is tips to lift your spirits. I like **E, M, O, V** and **U** best. I will practice the art of **E M O V U.**

E is for eat adventurously. You should try some new recipes. Buy different ingredients and pour some love into making food you really want to eat.

I will be adventurous, enjoying a warming soup on a not-so-warm day by the sea in my hut, heated on a little gas bottle powered stove. I've never had soup by the sea. I will boil water in my whistling kettle and pour steaming love into two mugs for a beverage, to be enjoyed with a choice of biscuits. Heaven.

M is for, make each moment count. Learn to savour the moment. This combines both mindfulness and gratitude, and is proven to boost your mental well-being. Notice the sights, sounds and emotions of each moment, and be grateful for the little things.

I'll be grateful for my little hut beside the seaside where I can enjoy the sight of seagulls soaring. The sound of happy children splashing in the sea, the crashing waves when the tide is in, and the crunching of pebbles as people pass by at a distance. The crunching of a tasty biscuit will be nice too.

O is for open book. Why not read that book that has been sitting beside your bed collecting dust for months. Make yourself a cuppa and curl up on the sofa, or take yourself to bed and completely immerse yourself in a good book. It's a great way to relax.

I will pop my whistling kettle on for a cuppa in my beach hut and sit comfortably in a festival chair with a new book. I'm tempted by one I saw advertised in *Weekly Wife* – *A Cornish Secret* by Emma Burstall, about the life, loves and secrets of a Cornish village by the sea. Hidden pasts surface in a message in a bottle. Intriguing.

U is for unleash your inner child. Focus on games that make you laugh.

I could play Monopoly, sitting on the decking with Ben. Or I spy, or hide and seek round the beach huts (maybe not). Or sit giggling together at the antics of dogs and children splashing about in the sea. Buy a bucket and spade and build a sandcastle. Instead of playing with dolls, I'll buy a small cast iron mermaid I liked in a gift shop at Dungeness a few years ago. There were quite a few in the shop, in different poses, and I hope there will still be some in stock. I'll take arty photos of her in the shallows, seaweed swirling around her tail, for my niece who loves mermaids.

V is for visions for the future. Vision boards are powerful things. Create a picture – physical or mental – of where you want to be and what you want to be doing in three, six or twelve months.

I want to be in my beach hut sometime this summer, hopefully June. And when it's renovated later in the summer, playing Monopoly on my decking with Ben. Me, with a get-out-of-jail-free card and landing on one of the posh properties like Park Lane and buying it. And trying not to lose the dice in the pebbles when I accidentally throw them off the decking.

5.00 p.m.   Bill and Ben, my beach hut men, will be meeting Andrew about now.

5.26 p.m.   I wonder how their meeting is going.

6.00 p.m.   I hope it's going well.

6.25 p.m.   I can't eat until I know everything is alright, and they are happy with what they find.

7.00 p.m.   I wish I knew what was happening.

7.22 p.m.   Maybe Ben wants to break bad news to me gently when he gets home.

7.30 p.m.   I can't eat. I'll just nibble a piece of toast. It could be a while before Ben comes home. It'll take about an hour to drive Bill back to Hastings. Then they will probably have a meal there or a pizza at a place they like in Rye. After that Ben will have to drive Bill home, where he'll have a coffee, before the hour's journey home.

I see in TV Weekly, *Escape To The Château: DIY* is on at 8 o'clock. But I can't watch it, I'll be worrying that the DIY needed for the beach hut may not be do-able. *DIY SOS: The Big Build* is on later. I like Nick Knowles. Him and his team are so amusing but that will be a no-watch too. Maybe I'll watch *Portrait Artist Of The Year* and admire the wonderful use of colour and light, unique use of brushwork, daring use of bold colours and fabulous technique – such vim and vigour – the colours full of vitality. And feel ever so envious that I'll never be able to paint like that. So I think I will watch *Agatha Christie's Marple* instead. That'll cheer me up nicely.

8.31 p.m.   Ben sends me a text message:

ON WAY HOME – HUT BONE DRY – DIY DOABLE – LATE VIEWING
COZ ANDREW GOT HELD UP

8.32 p.m.   I reply:

HURRAH – SAFE JOURNEY HOME X

Wednesday 11th

7.36 a.m.   I wake up smiling, after pleasant dreams where I was sitting on the decking of my beach hut, laughing, drinking minty tea and playing Monopoly with a mermaid. She loved the colour of the tea because it reminded her of seaweed. I told her I used to take kelp tablets made from large, brown, very nutritious seaweed, and this impressed her because seaweed was her favourite snack. I also mentioned I use an organic face cream called Green Angel, made in Ireland from Irish hand harvested seaweed. She said she'd like to try it.

After our fun game the mermaid swam off for a fresh fish supper and I sat on my decking, happily watching her diving into the waves until her tail fin disappeared under the water.

I play Monopoly
With a mermaid by the sea
We're sitting on my decking
With a minty cup of tea

9.00 a.m.   Ben is still snoring. I have no idea what time he got home last night because I'd plodded off to bed early, to seaside dreamland. But I *very much* look forward to him telling me all about yesterday in Herne Bay.

62

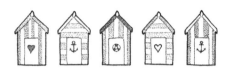

10.10 a.m.

ME: Thanks for checking out the hut yesterday.

BEN: No probs.

ME: I'm *so glad* it looks do-able.

BEN: Yeah. It's in a dry condition. But there was so much stuff in it, it was difficult to see what condition the units were in.

ME: What was in the hut, apart from the kayak?

BEN: Life jackets.

ME: No mouldy wetsuits?

BEN: Nope. Just mouldy towels, deckchairs, loungers, picnic chairs and tables....... erm....... windbreaks...... kids' beach stuff. Andrew said the owner didn't seem bothered about any of it.

ME: I expect he wants us to do a hut clearance.

BEN: I said we'd sort it.

ME: Oh yes, I remember you saying that to Andrew back in April. What happens about the paperwork?

BEN: There will be three sets of paperwork for you to sign. Andrew will send the details of the exact amount it will cost, including the council's ground rent. Then you will need to transfer the money to an account.

ME: Do you know which account?

BEN: The beach hut holding account. The money stays there until all the paperwork is signed and with him. Only then does he give you the deed of ownership and the beach hut owner the money. Like conveyance solicitors when you buy a house.

ME: Can't wait to sign!

BEN: You'll be dreaming about it.

ME: I dreamt I was playing monopoly on my beach hut decking with a mermaid.

BEN: You could design a seaside Monopoly.

ME: That's a thought. I could make a board for us. Instead of moving a little silvery top hat, dog, boot or battle-ship around the board, I could paint small seaside pebbles with a dolphin, shell or fish design.

BEN: A seagull or sandcastle.

ME: A mermaid.

BEN: You could land on *Sinking Ship* and have to miss two goes and pay the RNLI two hundred pounds. But be fine if you had a *Get Out Of Drowning* card.

ME: Land on *Shark Bay Waters* and have to pay lifeguards two hundred pounds. But be fine if you had a –

BEN: *Get Out Of Shark Attack* card.

ME: Landing on *Dolphin Bay* would mean you collect one hundred pounds and if you get a *Win A Mermaid Beauty Contest* card you get three hundred pounds.

BEN: Landing on *Treasure From Shipwreck* card, you receive seven hundred pounds!

ME: But only if have a *Get Out Of Drowning From Shipwreck* card. If you don't have that you'll be okay with a *Swimming With Mermaids* card.

BEN: And if you don't have either?

ME: You miss four goes, don't pass *GO,* collect two hundred pounds, or seven hundred pounds.

BEN: Instead of red plastic hotels and green plastic houses, we could have stripy red and white or green and white beach huts.

ME: Yes. Maybe one of our friends has an old Monopoly game they don't want anymore. I could paint white stripes on the little green houses and red hotels, and pretend they are beach huts.

2.26 p.m.   Ben returns from a lunchtime drink at The Ship Inn with his mate Rob, in a merry mood.

BEN: You could have pubs on your seaside Monopoly board. The Ship or The Jolly Sailor.

ME: Yes. Or The Neptune, like the pub on Whitstable beach, or the The Mermaid Inn where we've stayed many times in Rye.

BEN: Rob and I came up with a few ideas.

ME: Do tell!

BEN: You could land on *Jellyfish Bay* and get stung for one hundred and fifty pounds.

ME: Unless you had a *Get Out Of Jelly Fish Sting* card.

BEN: There could be a *Take A Trip To Herne Bay* card and if you pass GO collect two hundred pounds.

ME: And the same for a *Take A Trip To Whitstable* card.

BEN: Rob thought there could be a *Make Repairs On Your Beach Hut* card. For each green and white stripy beach hut – thirty pounds, and each red and white hut – one hundred pounds.

ME: Yes (cackling).

BEN: And you could have a card that said *Advance To Sandy Beach* and if you pass *GO* collect one hundred pounds. If you had a *Build A Sand Castle* card when you land on *Sandy Beach* you could get twenty-five pounds.

ME: And if you've got a *Deckchair* card you could get twenty pounds.

BEN: An *Ice Cream Cone* card, five pounds.

ME: A *Stick Of Rock* card, five pounds.

BEN: An *Ice Cream With A Chocolate Flake* card, ten pounds.

WE LAUGH

3.00 p.m.	I find dice in a drawer, full of bits and pieces.

ME: I've found dice we could use in the game, only half the size of your normal dice. They were in a Christmas cracker – look.

BEN: They'll be fine (smiling).

4.00 p.m.   I notice in TV Weekly, *Pirates of the Caribbean* is on later in the week.

ME: On my seaside Monopoly board you could land on *Ship Captured By Pirates* and have to pay one hundred pounds unless you have a *Defeat The Pirates* card. And if you land on *Smuggler's Cove* you get one hundred and fifty pounds for the sale of your contraband.

BEN: I can't wait to play the game now (laughing).

5.20 p.m.

ME: I've just been watching *Room 101*. That designer chap, Lawrence Llewelyn-Bowen, the actor Charles Dance, and a woman I've never heard of, were airing their views about their pet hates. It was quite funny when Lawrence was going on about how much he hated the colour beige, when used in interior design. The man presenting the programme, pointed out that Lawrence advertised his own beige furniture and a headboard in beige. Lawrence said it wasn't beige, it was camel! And was *most insistent*. I did cackle.

But what I'm getting around to telling you, is the

funny story Charles Dance told. Can't recall what he was complaining about, what his pet hate was. It was a story about Monopoly... Ah, I remember now, the woman I've never heard of was complaining about people who make up their own rules in Monopoly.

BEN: Wonder what she'd think of people who make up their own game of Monopoly, set at the seaside.

ME: Yes (smiling). Anyway, Charles Dance said he used to rent a flat in his drama student days with some mates. On Sunday they would play Monopoly and invite the landlord to join them, who would keep the money he got in the game, in lieu of rent.

BEN: Good story!

Friday 12th

10.00 a.m.   I make a start on the rewrite of the second chapter of my book, set in April. I can *now see* myself typing the final draft on my laptop, in my hut, like Roald Dahl writing away in a shed at the bottom of his garden.

Thursday 1st

8.40 a.m.

ME: *I saw my first bumble bee of the year today (spreading honey on toast). It was merrily buzzing around my head and had such a large fluffy body, I wanted to stroke it.*

BEN: *Would you like one for a pet?*

ME: *That would be very sweet.*

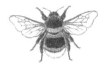

ME: *Wanda of Weekly Witch says bees remind us to stay focused on what is important and to smell the sweet nectar of life.*

BEN: *Is that why you're sniffing the honey jar?*

ME: *Of course. Did you know the ancient Greeks thought that honey was the elixir of the gods? According to their beliefs, the gods lived on Mount Olympus, consuming a diet of nectar and ambrosia, which made them immortal.*

BEN: *That was nice for them. I haven't had Ambrosia creamed rice pudding for years (licking lips).*

ME: *Shall I put some on tomorrow's shopping list?*

BEN: *Yeah.*

ME: *Zeus, the greatest of Greek gods, was raised on honey.*

BEN: *And Ambrosia creamed rice pudding?*

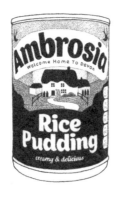

11.04 a.m.   *Knock! Knock! On our front door.*

BEN: *Who's there?*

ME: *It's for me.*

BEN: *How do you know?*

ME: *My witchy senses tell me.*

11.05 a.m.

ME: *It's my flowers (opening small brown jiffy bag).*

BEN: *Flowers? Invisible flowers are they?*

ME: *They're packets of seeds from www.prettywild-seeds.co.uk*

BEN: *Ah.*

ME: *A witch loves wild flowers as well as herbs in her* garden. And they will attract the butterflies and bees.

BEN: And fairy folk?

ME: Of course. The variety of flowers will look so pretty. And I can press a few petals to decorate candles for my spell work.

BEN: There isn't a photo on the packet of what the flowers will look like.

ME: Well, reading the variety of flowers, and I grew them in a cottage garden before I met you, they'll be lovely. Although one packet was a bit of a surprise.

BEN: Why was that?

ME: It came up celery.

BEN: Oh dear (laughing).

ME: There's a label on the back of the packet that names all the flower seeds. Quite a selection. I've counted twenty-one. I recognize a few – tansy, bird's foot, cornflower, corn poppy, corn marigold.

BEN: You may end up with corn on the cob!

ME: *Or celery again (cackling). Do you fancy sweetcorn*
           chowder with bread rolls with seedy bits in?

BEN: *Yeah. Will you add wild flower seeds to the rolls?*

ME: *It could bring a wonderful variety of colours to*
           our cheeks.

WE LAUGH

5.15 p.m.   I'm watching *Sun, Sea and Selling Houses,* and day-
            dreaming of sun, sea and a mini home that will be
            sold to me.

7.07 p.m.   *The Great Home Transformation* is on Channel 4,
            with Emma Willis and Nick Grimshaw, and I'm
            daydreaming of my own transformation of a negl-
            ected little hut into a mini, cosy haven.

9.16 p.m.   A couple have designed a contemporary, timber-
            clad kit house on *Grand Designs: The Streets,* with
            Kevin McCloud. I'm going to enjoy KitKats in my
            wooden hut, designed for comfort.

Saturday 14th

10.10 a.m.

ME: I've been thinking about my beach hut.

BEN: There's a surprise (smiling).

ME: I can't wait to see it again and pat the tired, sad, blue
           paintwork. It looked so gloomy – the huts either side

looking well, bright and nicely painted. I know it sounds silly, but I want to tell the hut we'll soon have it feeling better with a nice scrub down, new coat of paint, and a repair of the rusty hinges and locks, so it can move its doors more easily.

BEN: Like an old man who feels much better after a long, cleansing, warm bath, making his rusty old joints move more easily.

ME: And a new coat makes him feel good too.

BEN: On the subject of old men! Bill says we need a small set of steps, rather than a ladder for the painting. Make the job a lot easier. I'll get some in Wilko.

ME: That'll be lovely (gazing, at the garden, smiling). Do you know, it would usually make me sad, watching the bluebells wave goodbye to springtime in the breeze. But the thought of seeing my hut painted a beautiful bluebell-ish blue is making me really cheerful. And I'm looking forward to seeing Rob Bell later.

BEN: Who's he?

ME: The presenter of a programme about lighthouses. Part three is on tonight. He'll be visiting Longstone Lighthouse, off the coast of Northumberland. It's the spiritual home of lifesaving and the scene of a much discussed rescue attempt by the lighthouse keeper's daughter, Grace Darling.

BEN: I expect the lighthouse keeper used to say, 'Grace darling you're a lifesaver'.

ME: Yes (giggling). I think I'll get a little model of a lighthouse for my hut. Saw some lovely wooden ones when we were at the lighthouse in Dungeness a few years ago.

BEN: And you wished you could climb up the steps of the lighthouse and enjoy the view, like we did when we climbed the steps up to the bell tower in the church at he top of the hill in Rye.

ME: That was an *amazing view.*

BEN: Yeah. Pity the lighthouse had one hundred and sixty-nine steps.

ME: I feel a little faint with exhaustion at the thought of attempting to climb them.

BEN: I feel tired at the thought too.

ME: It must make someone of any age feel like they've achieved something, climbing *all those steps* and getting to the top.

BEN: And being rewarded with a fabulous view of the power station!

WE LAUGH

ME: Talking of achievements, I've been watching Steve Backshall in *Expedition With Steve Backshall.* You wouldn't believe the things he's done.

BEN: I'm sure you're going to tell me all about it.

ME: He's so brave. Goes on adventures to amazing, beautiful places on the planet where no man has gone before, and sees the most wondrous wildlife.

BEN: Good for him.

ME: Treks through dense jungle forest, explores dramatic underworld caves full of bats and snakes.

BEN: You'd love that.

ME: That I would!... He climbs vertical rock faces, wades through painful, glacial waters, risks being killed by an avalanche, and navigates *extremely dangerous, life-threatening* rapids full of crocodiles in a kayak.

BEN: Does Mr Backshall have a death wish?

ME: He said everyone asks him that. He always replies, no, he just has a lot of life! I've been feeling some energy coming back lately and kayaks do look lots of fun, so I can visualise myself paddling through rapids already, saying hello to the crocodiles.

BEN: Just because you'll soon be the owner of a kayak –

ME: And paddles, and a life jacket to keep me safe.

BEN: Doesn't mean –

ME: I can dream (smiling).

12.20 p.m. Time to stop daydreaming about sailing wildly down life-threatening rapids and drift back to completing the next chapter of my book – April.

Friday 2nd

ME: *Travel restrictions have come to an end today in the UK, as long as you stay in your bubble.*

BEN: *We'll stay in our hubble bubble. Me, my little witch and her two furry familiars, Diamanda and Lovely.*

ME: *And I do enjoy a bath full of witchy hubble bubble bath with lots of purple frothiness. I bought some for my not-so-little witchy niece for her birthday. She loves it.*

BEN: *It's your birthday soon. What do you fancy doing?*

ME: *Well, I do like to be beside the seaside on my birthday. But it'll be Easter weekend, so it's likely to be busy beside the seaside, now that travel restrictions are lifted.*

BEN: *Yeah. And showery weather is expected anyway.*

ME: *What I need is a little beach hut. In Whitstable or Tankerton.*

BEN: *Or Herne Bay.*

10.33 a.m.

ME: I hope the paperwork will arrive from the Herne Bay Beach Hut Association this week.

BEN: Is your pen poised ready to sign?

ME: It most certainly is.

BEN: I'm off now for my morning plod.

ME: It'll be good for you to have your morning walk along the beach when we go to the hut. Wendy of Weekly Wife said a study by the National Trust found that people sleep for forty-seven minutes longer on average, after a walk along the coast, compared to twelve minutes of extra sleep after an inland walk.

BEN: That's good to know.

ME: I've always noticed you sleep *much longer* after a day walking along the beach with Bill, when you visit him. Scientists have suggested this may be because the sea air is full of negative hydrogen ions.

BEN: She's off (laughing).

ME: These charged particles, abundant in sea spray and fresh air, improve the body's ability to absorb oxygen.

BEN: Marvellous.

ME: Yes. More oxygen can boost levels of the feel-good brain chemical serotonin, making us less prone to anxiety, so we get more shut-eye.

z z z z z z z z z

BEN: Close your eyes.

ME: Okay.

BEN: Both?

ME: Yes.

BEN: Hold out both paws close together.

ME: Okay... Oh my goodness, it's so heavy I can't hold it!

BEN: Open eyes.

ME: Wow! It's enormous. The biggest cauliflower I've ever seen. Forget about Steve Backshall and his achievements, it must feel quite an achievement to grow handsome veg. This must be the size of a football. I wonder how much it weighs.

BEN: I got it from the veg stall. The broccoli, tomatoes and carrots are impressive too.

ME: Yes. And they all look *very fresh* and delicious.

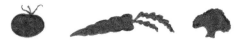

BEN: The cauliflower weighs just over five and a half pounds.

ME: Impressive. Wanda of Weekly Witch says cauliflower is one of the most healthy vegetables you can eat and supports the heart chakra, which is concerned with emotions. Wendy of –

BEN: Weekly Wife.

ME: Says it's a nutritional powerhouse, high in fibre, vitamins A, C and K, choline – which helps mood and memory. And quercetin, which can help the prevention of cancer.

BEN: We'll have lots of fresh cauli with dinner tonight.

ME: You are so beautiful, I just want to gaze at you for hours. I don't want to eat you, just enjoy your beauty (patting cauliflower on head). And you are very beautiful too (stroking Diamanda and Lovely on their soft heads, while admiring their nose and whiskers).

BEN: What about me?

ME: You have a beautiful nose and whiskers too dear (patting Ben on the cheek).

1.27 p.m.   I continue to work on the rewrite of my book. Still in April.

Saturday 3rd

12.45 p.m.

BEN: What are you up to?

ME: Just planning a bit of spell work (witchy glint in eye). It's the time of year to plant my wild flower seeds, but at the moment the weather feels February-ish. Peering into my crystal ball I see snow on the way.

BEN: Are you sure that's not just a fuzzy picture?

ME: Maybe. We'll have to wait and see. Anyway it'll be fun to give the seeds a little encouragement to grow with a little spell work. I'll begin by lighting a leafy-green candle to represent plants and growth, and a brown candle to represent the –

BEN: Earth.

ME: Yes. I have cornflower blue and poppy red scented candles too. A gift from you last Christmas, with pictures of flower fairies on, remember?

BEN: Amazingly I do!

ME: I'm sure I have a lavender scented candle too somewhere. This is going to be a most delightfully scented spell.

BEN: Any chanting involved?

ME: Of course. I'll sprinkle a small handful of wild flower seeds around the candles, envisaging scattering seeds in the garden, while honouring the sunshine and rain that will give them life and make them flourish.

BEN: And the fairies dance for joy...... Any singing?

ME: *I think I'll sing a cornflower fairy song, written by the fairy illustrator, Cicely Mary Barker. It starts:*

Mid scarlet of poppies and gold of the corn
In wide-spreading fields, the cornflowers were born
But now I look around me and what do I see?
That lilies and roses are neighbours to me!

❇ ❇ ❇ ❇ ❇ ❇ ❇

I'll sing her poppy fairy song too. It begins:

The green wheat's a-growing
The lark sings on high
In scarlet silk a-glowing
Here stand I

BEN: *Very nice.*

ME: *And the lavender fairy song is sweet, it begins:*

Lavenders blue, diddle, diddle
So goes the song

BEN: *I look forward to hearing the full versions.*

ME: *I could find my flower fairy book and sing you the songs now.*

BEN: *Maybe later. I'm off to meet my mate Les.*

Monday 16th

8.32 a.m.

ME: I dreamt last night that we were eating cauliflower cheese at my beach hut. Then I disappeared off into the sunset, rowing towards the horizon in my kayak, ending up in rapids in the Amazon with friendly crocodiles with big, toothy smiles.

BEN: No doubt you dreamt that, because we enjoyed a cauliflower cheese dinner late in the evening and you saw me ordering things on the Amazon website.

ME: Yes, I'm sure you're right. Maybe I'll have just one little go on the kayak before I sell it.

BEN: Not sure that's a good idea dear.

8.52 a.m.

ME: It's so dull, damp and chilly after a rainy weekend.

BEN: Yeah.

ME: I hope we're not going to have a dull, mostly rainy summer.

BEN: Why the grim face?

ME: I don't know. After feeding the wildlife, wet hedge leaves dripping on my face, I recalled a nightmare.

BEN: I thought you had a nice dream about cauliflower cheese and friendly crocodiles with toothy smiles.

ME: I did. But this was after. I was rowing along in my kayak under a blue sky, the same blue as I'm going to paint my hut, when huge, white cauliflower-shaped clouds appeared. They rained grated cheese and enormous, blue cheese sauce waves engulfed me, tossing me around like a salad in oil. I capsized and awoke enduring cold, mouldy cheese thoughts, that I wouldn't get to buy my hut for some reason.

BEN: Scrape the mouldy thoughts off your brain dear.

ME: Like brown spots off an old cauliflower?

BEN: Yeah. And enjoy a nice, relaxing hubble bubble bath.

ME: That I will do! Then get down to more rewriting.

10.26 a.m. I continue with the rewrite of *Saturday 3rd April*.

11.16 a.m.

ME: *The bells of St Michaels are peeling away.*

BEN: *Like me at Christmas with satsumas.*

ME: *Yes (cackling). I hope springtime sunshine will shine down on the happy couple and smiling guests.*

BEN: *So they have a cracking time, like you with walnuts at Christmas.*

ME: *There won't be many guests though, a maximum of fifteen is allowed at the moment. I expect a lot of weddings will be cancelled until next year.*

BEN: *It'll be a good excuse for a change of heart.*

ME: *Got a joke for you. Two TV ariels got married. The wedding was awful but –*

BEN: *The reception was brilliant.*

ME: *You've heard it!…. I do hope my little niece will find true love with the man of her dreams. She will be a most beautiful bride.*

11.a.m.   I hear the tap, tap, tap of the post arriving through the letter box and hurry as fast as my little paws will carry me, to the front door…… Will it be?……. Is it?…… The paperwork for my beach hut?……… No, not yet.

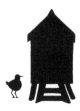

Tuesday 17th

7.17 a.m.   Nick Kershaw is singing on Radio Kent:

I won't let the sun go down on me
I won't let the sun go down

The presenter, Julia, said the song was apt because

the weather will be be very sunny today – it's going to be the hottest day of the year so far. Things will be looking up, when the sun comes up.

8.46 a.m.

ME: I hope Andrew has posted my beach hut paperwork.

BEN: There may be a large envelope winging its way to you.

ME: Towards the shore of our little street. The lapping waves of letterboxes. Soaring in my direction like the seagulls in Herne Bay, swooping and squawking – Sign me! Sign me! Sign me!

BEN: What are you like.

ME: I may be like a naive person. Andrew *did* say it would all take a while. What's a while?...... Weeks? Months? .... My payment for the hut was transferred to the Beach Hut Association last week, with the council tax. So I'm already paying tax on the hut, but I can't get in there yet. I do hope I'm not kept waiting till the end of this summer. Will there be a lovely, long spell of sunny weather with an opportunity to paint the hut, but I finally get *THE KEYS* when the rains come again. Will we just sit in the hut when I get the keys, surrounded by paint tins and paint brushes, while the rain falls? Instead of paint splashes on jeans, will it be just watching waves splashing on the shore?

BEN: Have a relaxing, witchy hubble bubble bath dear.

ME: I will. And I'll not hover by the front door tomorrow like a wee doggie, eagerly waiting to grab the post with my teeth as it shoots through the letterbox. I will get on with the rewrite of my book.

11.06 a.m.   I continue writing *Saturday 3rd April*.

1.36 p.m.   *I received a text message from my niece:*

HI AUNTIE, THANX FOR MY EASTER BUNNY CARD – WUD
YOU MIND SENDING ME A SPELL TO FIND TRUE LOVE ?

1.38 p.m.   *I reply:*

OF COURSE I CAN MY DEAR LITTLE WITCH – MUCH OF A
GOOD WITCHE'S WORK IS HELPING OTHERS – IT IS MOST
FUN WHEN IT IS FOR FAMILY XX

1.40 p.m.   *Louise replied:*

COOL – THANX AUNTIE XX

2.00 p.m.   *I consulted my spell book and found one I liked, to find true love.*

2.07 p.m.   *Found my best witchy writing paper and black felt-tip pen – best for writing curly italic spell writing, with lots of love and best witches.*

Dear Louise

Here's a little spell to help you find true love. I will send you some of the things you need.

Six green buttons

Green wool

Rose-scented oil

I have a green cardigan that I no-longer wear, I can take the buttons off that. I also have olive green wool and rose oil. Lastly you will need a rose in a vase. I thought you could borrow one from the bouquet I sent your mum for her birthday.

At sunrise (you'll have to get up early), thread the six green buttons onto the piece of green wool. Green is the sacred colour linked to Venus – the Roman mythological goddess of love and romance.

Tie the ends of the wool together to make a circle of about 13cm across. Then take a couple of strands of your lovely blonde hair out of your hair brush and tie them into a circle. Place the circle around the bottom of your vase that holds your rose. Your dad has made lots of little pottery vases, so you could use one of those! Next, pour a drop of rose-scented oil onto your hands, sniff, and chant:

Lady of green, from high above, send to me the power of love. With this circle here entire, send to me on wings of fire, a vision from a heart confined, that to my worth I am not blind, and so a TRUE

LOVE I can find.

Let me know when you are doing the spell and I will light a pink candle at the same time.

Happy spell work!

Love & Best Witches

Auntie xxx

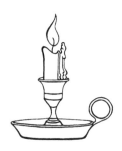

Monday 23rd

10.10 a.m.

ME: No sign of papers to sign for the hut yet. I hope there isn't a problem. It's been raining *so much,* is it going to rain all summer? Will it be hard to find a day you can paint the hut? Will we get freezing weather in June? We did get snow in April.

BEN: Yeah, you saw it in your crystal ball.

ME: That I did. Wasn't just a fuzzy picture, full of white flakes!

11.36 a.m. I hear tapping sounds coming from the letterbox.

ME: Just a clothes catalogue, gift catalogue, and a couple of flyers for pizza and Indian food. Not one paper to sign. My stars in Weekly Wife say it's a frustrating time. A restless stretch, during which I will find it hard to focus on one activity.

BEN: Have a hubble bubble bath dear.

ME: I will. Then I'll get down to more rewriting of April. The fourth begins with text messages and a letter to my niece, with recipes, so shouldn't take much focusing or concentration.

Sunday 4th

10.21 a.m. *I receive a text message from Louise:*

HI AUNTIE, THANX FOR THE EASTER CHOC BUNNY UNCLE LEFT IN OUR PORCH - IT IS CUTE - CAN'T WAIT TO GET YOUR SPELL TO BRING ME TRUE LOVE XXX

10.23 a.m. *I reply:*

GLAD YOU LIKED YOUR CHOC BUNNY LITTLE WITCH - THE SPELL TO BRING YOU TRUE LOVE WILL SOON BE ON ITS WAY TO YOU - FLUFFY EASTER BUNNY HUGS XXX

11.06 a.m. *I found The Real Witches' Kitchen and my witchy writing paper, then settled down to writing another letter to Louise.*

Dear Louise

As you've been enjoying baking during the pandemic, I thought you would like to make seed cake. It was popular during Victorian times, and is delicious, thinly sliced with a hot cuppa. Here's the recipe:

Seed Cake

Ingredients:

175g butter, softened (¾ cup)

175g caster sugar (very scant cup, less about 2 TBS)

3 large free range eggs, beaten

3 tsp caraway seeds

225g plain flour, sifted (1 ½ cups plus 1 TBS)

1 tsp baking powder

pinch salt

1 TBS ground almonds

1 TBS milk

Preparation:

Preheat the oven to 180°C/350°F/gas mark 4. Butter and line a 2 pound loaf tin with baking powder. Set aside.

Cream together the butter and sugar until light and fluffy. Beat in the eggs, one at a time. Sift together the flour and baking powder. Stir this in along with the salt, almonds, seeds and milk. Mix well to combine evenly. Scrape into the prepared baking tin.

Bake for 45 to 55 minutes, or until well risen, golden brown and a toothpick inserted in the centre comes out clean.

Allow to cool completely in the tin. Store in airtight container. Cut into slices to serve.

Happy cooking!

Love & Best Witches

Auntie xxx

P. S. I saw a recipe for a Honey Cake, and I know you love honey so I thought you may like to make it.

Honey Cake

Ingredients:

5 large eggs

165g brown sugar

85g honey

65g wholemeal self raising flour

100g sliced almonds

Preparation:

Beat the sugar and honey into eggs until very thick. Then slowly stir in the flour and almonds (save some almonds for later). Pour into cake tin. Bake in a pre-heated oven at 180° C for 40 minutes. Let cake cool in tin.

2.00 p.m.   I leisurely peruse Cotton Traders clothes catalogue, admiring the bright summer fashions. A laughing model looks like she is perched on the banister of a beach hut. She is holding a slice of watermelon with a bite out of it, which looks a little ridiculous, because she's wearing white, linen-blend cropped trousers that could easily get melon drips on them. Although the melon colours *do* match the stripes in her top, so look good for the photo. I imagine a photo-shoot make-up person or photographer took a bite out of the melon for her, passed it to her and told her to be careful, and that is why she's laughing so much.

I like the navy and white, long sleeved tee-shirt on the next page. It would look good with my white leggings (that I would not eat a watermelon without a plate, while wearing). The along-the-boardwalk navy slip-ons with white laces and gold-tone eyelets, would match the top *and* the navy and the white striped mugs I'm taking to the hut when it's decorated. *When* I get the keys.

In the gift catalogue, I admire the deco lady shelf sitters – recalling the fashion plates of the 1920's, as more emancipated ladies were taking to the water in newly created navy and white striped bathing suits and bathing caps to match.

The paper-straw Deauville navy and white striped visor with bow detail at the back (and matching scarf) brings to mind ladies on a beach, sunning themselves by the art deco hotel they are staying at on the set of *Agatha Christie's Poirot – Evil Under The Sun*.

5.30 p.m.   Hailstones are drilling into the world outside. The sky darkens. Thunder rumbles in the heavens.

ME: I'm envisaging sitting, cosy in my hut, watching storm clouds approaching..... rolling towards the beach from the horizon...... then the rain crashes onto the pebbles as rolling waves splash onto the shore..... Later the sun appears and sparkles on the pebbles, making the pebbly colours shine. And I emerge to a wonderfully peaceful beach because everyone has gone home.

BEN: And you do a little witchy dance between the breakers, celebrating the healing power of nature.

ME: It'll be more of a little wiggle for two seconds.

BEN: Breaker dancing.

ME: Yes (cackling).

Tuesday 24th

3.33 p.m. Pottering in the attic, I found a very old book, *The Witche's Cookbook*. I had forgotten all about it. The heavy, dusty tome, with a midnight blue and purple cover, sprinkled with silvery stars and silhouettes of flying bats, looked magical. Under the title, written in beautiful, ornate gold lettering, was an illustration of a cauldron full of a bubbly, green broth, the green bubbles rising into the air.

I slowly and reverently turned the biscuit coloured pages – smelly, covered in age spots, and a little frayed at the edges, like some old witches I've met. But full of wickedly-delicious, witchcraft-inspired recipes, and knowledge – like many other witches I've met.

I noticed quite a few recipes I thought my niece would like to try. I may send them to her now, instead of writing them in my witchy book. Haven't decided. But I have decided to try out a couple myself, to take my mind off waiting for the beach hut papers to arrive.

4.04 p.m.

BEN: I'm off into town in a minute, want anything?

ME: Well, when I was in the attic earlier and –

BEN: I heard you clonking about.

ME: I came across *this* beautiful, old cookbook.

BEN: It looks witchily-magical.

ME: You *can* judge this book by its cover!.... I'd like to try some of the more simple recipes. *Toadstool Toppers* look tasty. It says here:

             Often found nestled in enchanted forest among the magical moss-lined groves, mushrooms emit powerful auras and can enhance your powers of intuition and provide a deep connection to the fae and gnome folk – the fungus attracts them!

BEN: I'm sure it does. Write me a list.

ME: We've got plenty of garlic, onions, red peppers, salt, ground black pepper, and my home-grown parsley for garnish. Just need button mushrooms, cream cheese and cheddar cheese.

BEN: My mouth's watering already.

ME: Mine too. I like the sound of the *Crow Familiar Nests.*

BEN: They look good.

ME: It says here:

Familiars are spirits who can possess living things like cats, dogs and crows. Crows make excellent familiars due to their intelligent nature and maternal instincts. Make the nests to commemorate your wise winged companions.

BEN: You've got plenty of 'em. And your furry feline companions.

ME: That I have..... I only need three ingredients for the crow nests. Angel-hair pasta and parmesan cheese to garnish, which we've got. Just need marinara sauce, whatever that is. I don't know if you can get it in this country, the book is American.

BEN: I'll look online.

ME: That'll be good. There's also a couple of other ingredients I'd like you to see if you can find online too, because I want to send send recipes to Louise and I'm not sure they are available in this country.

BEN: What are they?

ME: Firstly, dragon fruit.

BEN: My sister-in-law grows it in her garden in the Philippines.

ME: Oh yes, I remember. I wished you'd brought some home with you, when you last visited. I've never seen it in this country. It's in a recipe for a love potion – not to find love, but to give to a loved one for a gift. My niece has a nice boyfriend, so I think she may like to make this potion, to give to him. The book says, the ingredients you need are: frozen dragon fruit, frozen strawberries, raspberries, cherries and pomegranate, beetroot and rose water. All blended together, they make a delicious, glowing, red drink.

BEN: Sounds very fruity. What's the other ingredient you want me to find?

ME: Purple potatoes.

BEN: Never heard of them.

ME: Neither have I. They are in a recipe for *Intuitive Purple Potato Salad.* We've got avocado, onions, and mustard. Paprika, salt, pepper and parsley. Just need apple cider vinegar and the potatoes. It says here:

In witchcraft, the colour purple is most associated with the third eye chakra, i.e., your psychic abilities like intuition. Your intuition is the guiding light that tells you what you know in your heart to be true. Potatoes promote image magic and enhance spiritual awareness. When you're in need of clarity, this seemingly simple salad will help you open your eyes, all three of them.

BEN: I reckon purple carrots, cauliflower or cabbage will do instead. Or all three, to open all three eyes. If you can't get the spuds here.

ME: Yes, my witchy intuition tells me you are right!

BEN: Right, I'm off.

ME: Hang on, I'll write your list.

5.44 p.m.

BEN: You can get frozen dragon fruit in this country and at least one supermarket sells it – it's imported. Waitrose have them. Come and look at the screen.

ME: Oh yes, they call it speciality exotic fruit. I remember you showing me a photograph of it, that you took when you were in the Philippines. I can see why it's called dragon fruit, the yellowy-green leafy bits shooting out of the fruit, do look like flames shooting out of a purple dragon's mouth.

BEN: You can get (scrolling) marinara sauce in a jar, in Tesco.

ME: Ah, it's a tomato, pasta sauce. Will be tasty in pasta crow nests, topped with Parmesan.

BEN: And no doubt garnished with a sprig of parsley, artily placed.

ME: Last time you were in France, you brought back a lump of nice, smelly cheese, that reminded me of Parmesan. Just noticed we are very low on it, so maybe you could just pop over to France and get another nice, smelly lump.

BEN: Certainly milady.

WE LAUGH

ME: Did you find purple potatoes online?

BEN: Yep. They are available in a couple of varieties that grow in the UK, but not common by the look of it.

ME: Never mind. As you said, other purple veg will do, maybe cooked with our usual spuds...... Fancy tasty *Toadstool Toppers* tonight?

BEN: Yeah!

Thursday 26th

9.07 a.m.

BEN: After you'd gone to bed last night, Andrew emailed a form for you to sign, but I can't print it out because the printer isn't working. I think I'll pop over to see the beach hut owner today and pick up the form. He's signed his part.

ME: Where does he live?

BEN: Not far – near your sister, in Rainham.

ME: Oh good. That'll be lovely. Thank you! Things are sailing along nicely now.

9.17 a.m. I smile as I drift into the garden to feed the wildlife – the wind billowing my sails beautifully.

10.17 a.m. I smile as I navigate my way through the sitting room and back room to the kitchen, to switch the kettle on for a minty, seaweed-green cuppa.

10.27 a.m. It's both my hands on deck to do the washing-up, then fish plates and cutlery out of the bowl of hot water to rinse under the cold tap.

11.38 a.m. I pick up a jewellery catalogue that plops through the letterbox, and smile again because I'm not disappointed by the post today. I will soon have my first form to sign.

1.37 p.m.   I splash about in the bath like a joyful mermaid in the ocean.

3.17 p.m.   I'm tempted by a seahorse pendant in Pia catalogue – a silvery seahorse, starfish, scallop and puka shell on a chain. The mermaid's treasure earrings are delightful too – small, sterling silver scallops with a freshwater pearl. Will resist temptation.

3.18 p.m.   I'm *very, very* tempted by the pewter beach hut key ring. The catalogue says it has nostalgic charm – to hold onto memories of days beside the seaside.

That will do for me
And be ready for a key
I do believe I'm feeling
Almost moved to poetry

3.20 p.m.   I find a pen and start to fill in the catalogue form. As I'm about to complete it Ben strolls in through the front door.

BEN: I see you have a pen, poised ready in your hand. Ready to sign?

ME: That I am!

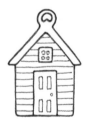

BEN: Here you are, the first of the paperwork requiring your signature madam.

ME: Thank you kind sir.

BEN: Andrew said you should get the next lot after the Bank Holiday.

ME: That might take a while. Thursday today. So they may arrive next Tuesday or Wednesday. But it'll probably be after that, because of the Queen's jubilee celebrations the following days. So maybe the week after that. I know I should be patient, but Cosmic Colin in Weekly Witch, said Mars is now joining with Jupiter, giving me more energy. This also means my patience will be in short supply.

BEN: I'll get you some patience in Sainsbury's. What do you fancy?

ME: Eggs and cottage cheese are calming foods.

BEN: Okay (laughing).

ME: Look at this photo of what I've just ordered from the Pia catalogue.

BEN: Perfect (laughing again).

ME: It will look even better with keys on it.

BEN: The man you're buying the hut from is a very nice old chap, Jerry.

ME: I *so feel* for him losing his wife.

BEN: They must have had happy times at the hut with their family. He said at one point, four generations were using it. They had it for twenty years.

ME: That's lovely.

BEN: He was *really pleased* you're keeping the painting of the sun on the roof. It meant a lot to him because his late wife Elizabeth painted it. She was an artist and went to the same art college as you!

ME: I knew as soon as I saw the hut that a creative, spiritual person had spent time there, and that it was the one for me. The posh, stripy one, that we never got a reply from, wasn't *really me*, too full of cupboards, and too expensive!

BEN: Yeah. Oh, and Jerry said it was lovely to know the hut was going to such a nice couple.

ME: That's good to know. Cuppa? (wiping away a happy little tear).

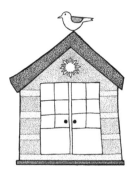

Chapter Three

June

Friday 10th

2.00 p.m.

ME: What a beautiful day! A perfect day to be here beside the seaside.

BEN: And you do like to be beside the sea.

ME: The warm sunshine and soft, cool summer breeze feels *so lovely* on my face.

BEN: Peaceful.

ME: Yes. We're so used to the constant rumbling and swishing sound of traffic. Shouting and screaming families and barking dogs on the low income estate.

BEN: Here, it's just the gentle rippling sound of waves as the tide goes out.

ME: And ripples of laughter from our beach-hut-but-one neighbours.

BEN: Friendly bunch!

ME: It was really nice when they called out hellos, with lots of smiles when we arrived earlier.

BEN: We're going to enjoy it here.

ME: And I'll love working on my book here too. The sea breeze clearing my mind. Little rippling waves of inspiration splashing onto my brain.

BEN: *Revitalising!.....* Will creativity flow like filigree foam, washing over the sandy shore of your mind?

ME: To be *shore*, to be *shore* (best Irish accent).

WE LAUGH

ME: It'll be lovely when we eventually get *the keys* and we can get inside the hut. I feel a bit silly sitting here, perched on the decking. But it's been sixteen days since I got the first paper to sign and –

BEN: You just couldn't wait to be here again.

ME: I'm glad I brought some cushions to sit on.

BEN: Think I'll go for a wander (getting up and rubbing back).

ME: Are you going to wander lonely as a cloud?

BEN: No, Mrs Wordsworth (laughing).

ME: Will you wander *lovely* as a cloud then, in your grey and white shirt?

BEN: Yeah!..... I'll leave you to your cloud watching.

ME: Not many clouds about today. I heard a very interesting programme on Radio Three last night about clouds and how they form. I was surprised at how fast they sometimes travel. Today the clouds are wispy – cirrus clouds. They are formed when warm, dry air rises, causing water deposition onto rocky or metallic dust particles at high altitudes. You wouldn't believe how high they are!

BEN: I'm sure you will inform me. But I'm off now for a plod.

2.04 p.m. I gaze up at wispy cirrus clouds, drifting thousands of meters above sea level in the June blue, making me feel as calm and high as being in love........ I see the wings of an angel.......... a dolphin with a very long snout........ a seahorse floating on its back....... Then watch Ben crunching his pebbly way down to the water's edge, lovely as a cloud in his grey and white shirt. A lone seagull, wearing similar colours, silently glides and circles only a few metres above sea level, then over his head.

As I watch Ben wandering, I come over all Wordsworth.

He wanders lovely as a cloud
In his grey and white old shirt
Admiring a young lady
In a pretty yellow skirt

I sit and wonder if William Wordsworth recited his poetry to his wife, Mary, in need of her opinion. Maybe he did. And after many years of hearing how beautiful the green linnet is, beneath the fruit tree boughs that shed snow-white blossoms on his head and how glorious daffodils are beneath the trees, fluttering and dancing in the breeze, as she grows older –

She wanders to the kitchen
To cook and crash and clatter
As he raises his voice in verse
And continues so to natter

He knew he was a great poet
So it didn't really matter

And he so loved a filling meal
Of sausages and batter

I can see him sitting on a beach with Mary, reciting the third verse of his poem about daffodils, that just came to him that morning.

The waves beside them danced; but they
Out-did the sparkling waves in glee
A poet could not but be gay,
In such jocund company

Mary gets up and wanders off, leaving him to be gay and poetic on his own.

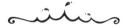

Like the seahorse cloud formation I saw in the sky, made of water vapour, resting its back on metallic dust particles, I rest my back against the hut door. I touch the decking – touching wood that I would receive more paperwork to sign soon. Then I smile, because I'm starting to feel at home here. I made the right decision.

I smile again as I notice an elderly couple, their trousers rolled up, enjoying a paddle in the shallows. Their golden Labrador bounces playfully around them, madly wagging its tail. They laugh a lot and pat the dog. I pat peeling, white paintwork on a banister and a rusty hinge (weeping a yellow stain), telling the hut not to cry and reassuring it that I will soon have it smiling again. It will soon (weather permitting) be nicely painted and happy like the huts on either side – the one on the left, a warm orange with Naples yellow veranda and the one on the right, a refreshing sea-green with white veranda.

2.07 p.m.   I decide to take a pebbly plod down to the waters edge to join Ben. It doesn't look far. Quite a short distance. BUT it doesn't feel quite so short when you don't realise until you are on your way, that the journey down to the waters edge is a few, fairly steep slopes and you keep almost falling over and walking a wobbly sideways walk, feeling *most self-conscious* that anyone watching (feels like the whole of Herne Bay) will think you are tipsy – that you've had too many glasses of wine with lunch. But like the explorer Steve Backshall, you enjoy a challenge. Although unlike Steve, you are not in danger of being eaten by a crocodile, crushed under an avalanche, almost drowned in rapids or falling off a vertical rock face. But you may fracture an ankle or a wrist, or break your nose when you fall, flat on your face onto the pebbly beach.

ME: Did you see me nearly fall over a few times?

BEN: No.

ME: I'm not used to walking on pebbly slopes. It's a bit like trying to walk down a cobbled street wearing high heeled shoes.

BEN: I wouldn't know about that.

ME: I must have looked like a very tipsy crab, wobbling sideways.

BEN: You can be a little crabby at times.

ME: Thanks!

BEN: Only joking dear.

ME: When we get back to the hut, would you mind asking me if I'd like a mineral water opened, nice and cold from the cool box – in a fairly loud voice, so the neighbours can hear?

BEN: Okay, why?

ME: So the neighbours won't think I had too much to drink at lunch.

BEN: They'll just think you are sobering up.

ME: Do you think so?

BEN: No (laughing). Oh, I forgot to mention, got an email from the beach hut owner, Jerry. He said his son is going to remove the kayak from the hut, and some of their belongings.

ME: That's a relief. I think I'd have got a bit weepy if I saw all their belongings, like the towels hanging on the wall, waiting for the family to return. *And* it'll save us the job of selling the kayak and transporting it.

BEN: And having loads of stuff to take to charity shops.

ME: If there's deckchairs and loungers left, maybe some of our fellow Herne hutters may like them, if they're not rusty. We prefer our festival chairs and old lounger.

BEN: Yeah we do. I met the lady who owns the hut next door to yours, on the right (pointing back up the beach), when I came to view the hut with Bill. She said she had inherited it and was just finishing painting doors.

ME: It does look good. Bright and fresh.

BEN: She was a very nice, friendly middle-aged lady.

ME: That's another relief, after all the bad neighbours we've had over the past ten years.

BEN: And I discovered the public loos. Clean and only a short walk. They are in part of the angler's club-house, and hidden around the side.

ME: Oh good. That'll be *another relief* a bit later.

BEN: I'll show you where they are before *we go*.

ME: I love all the different colours of the huts, especially the stripy ones – powder blue and white, violet and cobalt blue, poppy red and white.

BEN: I like the dark green.

ME: That's viridian.

BEN: And the dark blue and white stripes look good.

ME: It's marine blue and cream.

BEN: The dark pink is nice.

ME: Magenta.

BEN: If you say so dear.

WE LAUGH

ME: I love the way some people have been creative, decorating the roof or doors of their huts with shell designs. A heart, a seahorse or a seabird.

BEN: I expect, over time, when you're up to it, you'll be painting little fish designs on the sides or back of the hut. Or smily whales or mermaids.

ME: Sailing ships, shells or starfish.

BEN: Do you feel a Wordsworth moment coming on?

ME: Maybe....... I'd quite like my hut to be stripy but that would be a lot of work for you and Bill, and I'm happy with what I've decided.

BEN: Phew (wiping brow).

ME: *Shells and starfish*
Fishes and whales
Dolphins and seagulls

BEN: *And ships without sails*

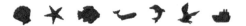

BEN: Just heard from Andrew.

ME: Is everything okay?

BEN: He's emailed the last of the paperwork for you to sign. I'll see if I can get the printer working.

ME: Oh lovely!

Wednesday 15th

10.44 a.m. I'm watching *A Place In The Sun* on Channel 4. A couple have found a property they love in Spain with a view of the sea. Many couples, searching for a home in Spain, desire a sea view. But sometimes the only place they can afford has just a small part-of-the-sea view in the distance. Or no view at all. I'm going to have a view, *the whole view, and nothing but the view!*

11.20 a.m. I browse through today's gift catalogue, admiring a white, wooden rocking chair.

ME: Look at this rocking chair. It would look lovely on my beach hut veranda don't you think?

BEN: Yes, very nice. You always wanted a rocking horse when you were were little, but couldn't have one. Now you're getting on in years and desire a rocking chair, you can have one. You could rock around the clock to your heart's content.

ME: Now you've said that, you know what Bill Haley song I'm going to have on my brain.

I'm gonna rock
Gonna rock around
The clock tonight!

BEN: I can see you gently rocking to the rolling waves on your veranda.

ME: I do like a bit of rock and roll.

I'm gonna rock
And enjoy my whole
Sea view today!

BEN: I like a bit of rock cake. They do a tasty one at the café on the pier.

ME: I like a *whole* rock cake. And a *whole* sea view. Nothing but the view.

BEN: I see myself in a festival chair enjoying a whole lot of picnic grub, piled high on one of our picnic plates.

ME: And whole mugs of steamy hot tea......... on second thoughts about the rocking chair, our festival chairs will be a lot more comfy than a wooden rocking chair, even with a nice, stripy cushion on the seat. Although rocking chairs *do look nice* on verandas.

BEN: I hear some verse coming on.

ME: I wonder if Mr Wordsworth's wife would say that to him, as they sipped their morning tea.

BEN: Yeah.

ME: *Rocking to the rolling sea*
As they sip their morning tea

BEN: Right, I'm off in a minute.

ME: Where?

BEN: Hastings. It's Bill's birthday.

ME: Oh yes, I remember now. Will you have a big, late lunch and not be wanting witchy soup with creepy croutons when you get home?

BEN: We're gonna have an early evening pizza at that place we like in Rye. We'll probably park at Pett Level, near the Winchelsea end, then walk to Rye along the coastal path, cutting up through the nature reserve to come out near Simply Italian restaurant, where we can sit outside for a G and T and pizza.

ME: Sounds really nice. And you have the perfect day for it. Got your hat and sun cream?

BEN: Yes dear.

11.22 a.m. I switch the kettle on for a minty cuppa and make up a little song.

We'll be sitting on the beach in June
I'll be going strong and so will you
We're gonna rock, gonna rock
With seaside rock tonight!

ME: Do you remember sugary, seaside rock. Pink or stripy with the words running all through the middle?

BEN: Yeah. I'm off now. See you later.

ME: Give Bill a birthday hug from me.

BEN: Will do.

11.45 a.m. I continue the rewrite of my book, which is coming along nicely. April done. I'm well into May now.

Wednesday 5th

10.42 a.m.   *I sent a text message to my niece:*

HI LOUISE, I'VE SENT YOU TWO RECIPES THAT I THINK YOU
WILL LIKE – THEY SHOULD ARRIVE SOON – AUNTIE X

11.12 a.m.   *Louise replied:*

OH YAY – CAN'T WAIT X

11.15 a.m.   *I sent another message:*

YOU KNOW THE CHARM BRACELET YOU LOVE? I READ IN
WEEKLY WITCH THAT CHARM BRACELETS TRADITIONALLY
BORE MAGICAL SYMBOLS THAT REPRESENTED THE WEARER'S
WISHES – SUCH AS A SUN FOR HEALTH AND A HEART TO
ATTRACT LOVE

11.17 a.m.   *Louise replied:*

I LOVE THE FAIRY CHARM YOU GAVE ME FOR XMAS – I DON'T
HAVE A SUN OR A HEART

11.18 a.m.   *I replied:*

NOW I KNOW WHAT TO GET YOU FOR YOUR BIRTHDAY IN
A FEW WEEKS AND I'VE SEEN A WITCHY HAT TOO X

11.20 a.m.   *I could see her sweet smile in my mind's eye as she
replied:*

CAN'T WAIT AUNTIE XX

6.00 p.m. Leafing through TV Weekly, I plan my evening's viewing. After *Coronation Street* I'll watch *Escape To The Château*. And I'll not wish I have a château to escape to – I will have a beautiful beach hut to escape to.

At 9.15 p.m. I'll watch *Best Of Britain By The Sea,* and will no-longer wish I was living on the Cornish coast next door to Dawn French. Will look forward to veggie Cornish pasty in my hut on the Kentish coast, next door to nice neighbours.

Drinking tea by the sea
Nautical mug on a coaster
Nibbling pasty instead of toast
Because I don't have a toaster

Friday 17th

10.04 a.m. Our shopping delivery arrives and Ben chats away to the young delivery man from ASDA.

ME: He sounded nice.

BEN: Yeah. He said if he knew we'd ordered asparagus he'd have given us some from his garden.

ME: That's sweet.

BEN: He said he fries it in butter.

ME: Sounds tasty. Fresh asparagus would have been lovely. Although I prefer it steamed, don't you?

BEN: Yeah.

ME: Today's delivery doesn't look fresh at all. The tips of the asparagus are a bit soft and going off. The ends are hard and woody. Ugh. The sprouts don't look good either. I'll need to peel the outer leaves, they look very brown and wrinkly in places.

BEN: Like an old, weathered witch, who has spent too much time riding her broomstick on hot, sunny days?

ME: Yes dear.

BEN: Do you feel a song coming on, to put in your witchy book, about old witches?

ME: Yes, I feel a song coming on, but not about witches. Inspired by rotting veg and a song I heard on Radio Kent this morning.

BEN: You're inspired by rotting veg? What's the song?

ME: It's from the sixties, by the Righteous Brothers – *You've lost that loving feeling.*

BEN: Lets hear it then. I'll work out the chords on my guitar.

ME: *You never close your eyes anymore*
When I kiss your lips
And there's no tenderness like before
In asparagus tips
I'm trying hard not show it baby
But baby, I know

          The sprouts are gonna need peeling

Oh, they will need a peeling
They will need lots of peeling
Now they're gone, gone, gone

BEN: *Almost gone right off!*

WE LAUGH

11.03 a.m.

ME: I expect the beach hutters will be making the most
         of the *huge heatwave* this weekend.

BEN: You mean Herne hutters.

ME: Oh yes. It's a week since I sent my signed paperwork
         to Andrew by email. I really hope we get the keys
         soon, my beach hut keyring is looking lonely without
         keys, and summer is ebbing away. Well, it will start
         to after Summer Solstice – the longest day of the
         year. I've been thinking, there may be constant rain
         after the heatwave and you won't get a chance to paint
         the hut for ages. And....

BEN: Chamomile tea?

ME: Mm, please. I read in Weekly Witch, chamomile is
         known as the flower of equilibrium. It's a symbol of
         energy and patience, and helps calm your nerves.

※   ※   ※   ❋   ※   ※   ※

BEN: We know about chamomile. Here you are, a calming
         brew for a witchypoo.

ME: Yes, but there are words you should say when brewing.

117

With bounteous hand and the
healthful balm, oh scentful
chamomile, most verdurous herb,
bring me health and heart.
Blessed be.

You must say this out loud next time you brew a chamomile tea. And in the moments before you drink the tea, if you share it with me, you should pause and enjoy the stillness. This will set the tone for the rest of your day, filled with a wonderful sense of well-being.

BEN: Anything you say dear. But I can't remember all that.

ME: I'll write it down.

BEN: I'm most obliged (laughing).

ME: Wanda of Weekly Witch has a good affirmation too.

My soul is connected to the
abundance of the universe. I am
ready to turn my dream into
a reality.

* * * ☽ ✺ 🪐 * * *

BEN: Now you have a *confirmation,* as well as an *affirmation.* Your dream is now a reality.

ME: You've not heard from, have you?

BEN: Yes, Andrew. The beach hut is now all yours.

ME: *Oh, wonderful!*

BEN: I'll email Jerry to find out when it's convenient to pick up the keys.

ME: *Lovely.* The presenter on Radio Kent said it's feel good Friday. And it most certainly is.

Tuesday 21st

8.00 a.m.

ME: What a glorious, almost Midsummer's Day morning. Druids are phoning into Radio Kent to say what they will be up to this Summer Solstice.

BEN: Will you be phoning-in to say what you are up to?

ME: I'll be tempted.

BEN: For a laugh!

ME: More a little cackle.

BEN: I know what you'll be doing. You'll be in the garden enjoying a bit of sun worship, wearing the colours of the festival. Maybe chanting in a whispery, witchy way.

ME: And as I think of the sun, our life giving star, I will look forward to the sun design on my beach hut being brought back to life with a coat of bright yellow paint.

BEN: You'll be lighting candles, the colours of the festival.

ME: And looking forward to light, bright sunny days beside the seaside.

BEN: Cooking food with the colours of the festival, using orange and red peppers. And yellow sweetcorn.

ME: And looking forward to taking salad with crunchy, colourful peppers in a Tupperware box, to the hut for lunch.

BEN: Texting your witchy niece to ask what she is doing for Summer Solstice.

ME: Looking forward to completing the final pages of the rewrite of my witchy diary, ready to type in my hut. Although I think I may finish it today.

BEN: Will you be using the black ballpoint, witchy pen I got you at the weekend, for inspiration?

ME: Oh yes! The Harry Potter pen. I like the little plastic talking hat on the end.

BEN: It's bendy, so you can make it do the movements the hat does in the film when it speaks. Though I don't suppose you do that.

ME: Noo (grinning). I've been using it to do some sketches for my book, it flows nicely.

BEN: The pen or the inspiration?

ME: Both!

BEN: Oh good, can I see them?

ME: Hang on.

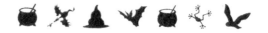

BEN: I like the cauldron and owl, the hats and the bats, frogs and the dragon, but where are the cats?

ME: You sound very poetic. Do you feel some verse coming on?

BEN: Not today.

ME: There will be a cat or two, maybe on a broomsick – I mean broomstick.

BEN: Is broom sickness the same as car sickness?

ME: Probably!

BEN: Did you notice, every time you click the pen on and off, little messages appear in the window in the side of the pen, the same dialogue as the talking hat in the Harry Potter film?

ME: Not at first. But when I did, it made me cackle when I read them.

Where shall I put you?
RAVENCLAW
HUFFLEPUFF
Hmm difficult.
VERY difficult.
GRYFINDOR
SLYTHERIN

Young Harry Potter fans will love this pen.

BEN: And the old ones.

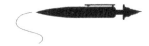

ME: I just heard a good joke on the radio. What's the best thing to put into a pie?

BEN: I don't know. Apples?

ME: Your teeth.

BEN: I fancy a pie now.

9.38 a.m.

BEN: I'm off for my morning plod. Will be popping into Sainsbury's. Want anything?

ME: A nice vegetarian pie. And a fruit pie for a treat. And there's something else we need, but I can't –

BEN: Text me when you remember.

ME: Will do.

1.36 p.m.

ME: Isn't that silver back gorilla gorgeous (pointing to TV screen).

BEN: Yeah, he is!

ME: You should come back as one in your next life.

BEN: Why?

ME: They are vegetarians and like to sit on vegetation, eating all day.

BEN: That'd suit me fine.

ME: Me too. I'd like to sit in my beach hut every day, all summer, feasting on delicious salads and pies. Crunching fresh, crispy lettuce, peppers and celery, like a big, hairy gorilla crunching on bamboo shoots and leaves, tree bark and wild celery, all day long.

BEN: I'd love to join you in your hut. I'm your big, hairy gorilla.

ME: That you are!

ME: There's a monkey, can't recall which breed, that has a good feed, then it stores food in a pouch in both cheeks so it can snack anytime it fancies. That would suit you too.

BEN: Yeah! I hear some verse coming on (hand to ear).

ME: *There was a monkey of some breed*
That would sit and have a good feed

BEN: *With a good book, enjoying a read*

ME: *Then store food in a pouch*
Then lie down on the couch

BEN: *Then get bitten by a flea*
And say ooh, ouch!

ME: The monkey storing food, brings to mind a work colleague who used to love to eat seedy bread rolls in her lunch hour, because the seeds stuck in her teeth, and she could enjoy a nibble as she worked at the drawing board after lunch!

2.07 p.m.

BEN: I saw you crawling on the lawn earlier. Were you pretending to be a gorilla or worshipping the sun?

ME: Neither. I was picking up bits of fairy garden ornament. She may have been knocked over by the foxes in the night when they came to feed. I could hear them. Their spooky, breathy bark is so eerie, especially on a moonlit night.

BEN: Can she be mended?

ME: Oh yes. I'll glue her wings back on.

BEN: Good. A fairy with broken wings is a sad sight.

ME: It's international Fairy Day on the twenty-fourth of June. It's a day to celebrate these little creatures of folklore. They are found in almost every culture in the world!

BEN: That's nice.

ME: To welcome the fae into your home and garden, you should leave offerings of fresh bread, honey and dried flowers.

BEN: So if I see you pottering at the bottom of the garden on Friday, I'll know you are leaving a gift for the fairy folk and telling them to –

ME: Come and get it!

3.00 p.m. I begin working on the rewrite of the final two pages of my book. It's Summer Solstice.

12.43 p.m. *I receive a text message from my niece:*

HI AUNTIE – THANX SO MUCH FOR THE RECIPES FROM WEEKLY WITCH – REALLY LOVED BAKING THEM – MUM AND DAD SAID THEY TASTED DELICIOUS XX

I replied:

YOU ARE MOST WELCOME LITTLE WITCH XX

1.04 p.m. *Louise sent me another text message:*

DID YOU GO OUT ON YOUR BROOMSTICK TO WATCH THE SUN RISE ?

I replied:

I DID – AND WILL FLY TO YOUR HOUSE THIS AFTERNOON TO DROP OFF SOME APPLES, A LARGE MAGICAL POTATO AND HERBS FROM MY GARDEN, SO YOU CAN MAKE THE WITCHY POTATO CAKES FROM A RECIPE I'VE SENT YOU – WHAT ARE YOU DOING FOR SUMMER SOLSTICE ?

Louise replied like a keen witch:

I'M WEARING THE COLOURS OF THE FESTIVAL – I DESIGNED A TEE-SHIRT WITH A RED, ORANGE AND YELLOW FLOWER USING THE FABRIC PENS YOU SENT TO ME, AND COOKING A PIZZA FOR MUM AND DAD WITH RED, ORANGE AND YELLOW PEPPERS

I replied:

THAT SOUNDS LOVELY − I LOOK FORWARD TO SEEING
YOU FOR A FLYING VISIT ABOUT 4 PM

Louise sounded happy and excited:

YAY − CAN-T WAIT XX

7.20 p.m.   After a tasty veggie pie and fresh veg, we enjoy delicious apple pie.

ME: I've written an ode to an apple pie.

BEN: Lets hear it then.

ME: *How I love you piece of pie*
You are the apple of my eye
But when you're gone
I will not cry

BEN: Because we can always have a pie treat again.

    Now you're gone I will want more
Next time, with custard I will pour

ME: *Your fluffy pastry so divine*

BEN: *Your golden beauty so sublime......* I remember the witchy apple pie you used to make!

WE LAUGH

8.10 p.m.

BEN: Just got an email from Jerry. I can pick up the beach hut keys on Thursday.

Monday 27th

1.03 p.m.   I'm sitting with a *big smile* on my face, on a small, round wooden table, found in the corner of my little hut. Enjoying the view. My *whole beach* view. Nothing but the peaceful view. A thousand times better than a wall of brickwork with the odd window, opposite our house, now that the new housing estate has been built. If it rains today, and I think it will soon, we won't have to hurry to the car.

While Ben enjoys his daily exercise, plodding along the pebbles to the pier for a coffee, I survey the contents of the hut. It's packed with quite a lot of stuff. A lot more than I thought there would be. And the more I sit, the smellier it seems to get. On closer inspection of the loungers – *very* rusty, *very* smelly.

Looks like there's four loungers, a chair and windbreaks, that will definitely not be suitable to offer to our beach hut neighbours or take to a charity shop. Ugh. I think Ben will need to book a dump trip or two. Or three, judging by all the clutter.

I thought I'd be sitting alone, feeling a bit tearful, looking at all the belongings that were left behind when the hut was closed up for the winter, waiting for the family to return when the weather turned warmer. And feeling sorrowful for the owner who had lost his wife after so many happy years – so many lovely times beside the seaside with their children, grandchildren and great-grandchildren.

But I'm not. I'm just a little sad. I think, because Jerry was so touched that I'm keeping the sunshine design on the hut roof, that his wife Elizabeth so lovingly painted. And I could feel her smiling in spirit world. I really could.

My heart smiles as I notice the children's seasidey things – buckets and spades, fishing nets, a frisbee (which brought back happy memories of playing frisbee with my dog) and all sorts. What fun they must have had, and they will always have the good beach hut memories.

Sipping mineral water, I look at the grubby kettle with the pile of stuff on the work surface, and think how nice it will be to have a little hob, powered by gas bottles. And a new kettle to make hot drinks. I'll buy a small saucepan to heat up soup on a chilly day too. And keep cuppa-soups in the cupboard.

I visualise myself, sipping tea and tapping away on my laptop, working on my book – now that it is all rewritten and ready to type away to my heart's content.

I really like the large mirror hanging on the back wall above the units. When all the piled up junk is removed, it will reflect the sea and sky. I'll have two views and the hut will feel bigger. It just needs a good clean and the frame given a lick of paint.

Staring at the part of the mirror I can see between the legs of a rather ugly plastic chair, I reflect how easy it will be to forget for a while, the awful things going on in our country and other countries, and just enjoy being here. Relaxing. Slowly breathing in and out. Like the tide.

I decide to explore, and gingerly open a cupboard. It is full. So is the other one. Full of stacks of mildew covered plates, plastic cups, china mugs, saucepans and all sorts. I don't want to rummage – they look dirty and slimy. I can't seem to open the cutlery drawer, which is just as well, I'm a little bit nervous that something is going to jump out at me. Will ask Ben, my strong gorilla man, to open it.

The stench starts to get too much for me. I begin to feel ill and wheezy – need to end my exploration and sit out on the decking and hope Ben returns soon, as it's going to rain. But I'm happy the hut will be lovely when everything has been removed and it is cleaned and repainted.

I notice a creepy-crawly on a seaside-themed clock with a picture of a camper van that I don't like at all, because it reminds of a rather unpleasant man in my past. That will have to go. I rescue the creepy-crawly with a piece of tissue from my pocket and place it gently on the pebbles near the decking.

A spider with big, scary legs, scuttles across the grubby, white wall, then stops as if watching me. I'm sure he's wondering who I am – I'm not who he was expecting. I apologize for the intrusion.

1.30 p.m.   Ben returns with a grin on his face.

BEN: Happy?

ME: Yes (smiling and picking up a frisbee). Did you know

a frisbee is named after the pie tins of the Frisbie bakery.

BEN: No. Where's the bakery?

ME: Bridgeport, Connecticut.

BEN: Fascinating.... I saw a chap repainting a few doors down from here. I said hello and asked if he had any advice or tips about renovating the hut. He said, no need to wash the outside of the hut, just give it a good brush and light sanding to make sure any loose bits are sorted, then use a good quality paint. A couple of coats will last longer on an older hut, especially if undercoated too.

ME: It's going to be perfect! And good as new when the rusty bits are sorted too. Some look like they need replacing.

BEN: As far as I can see, we'll need two side bolts with hoops for the padlocks and new cabin hooks and loops to hold the doors open. I'll contact the hut makers now.

1.33 p.m.   We perch on the decking, and it's not long before we hear from the hut makers.

BEN: The hut makers have replied and have replacement bolts and hooks in stock.

ME: Oh good.

BEN: They also confirmed, the hinges are stainless steel and should clean-up nicely with a cloth and bit of WD40 oil. There's a B&Q in Herne Bay. I'll take Bill there and we can get the rest of the things we need.

ME: Most of the stuff here is rusty and mildewy, you'll notice if you look closely.

BEN: Oh yeah.

ME: You'll need to book two or three dump trips I think, although there's a few things I'll save. Some can be cleaned-up, some painted. I'd like to go home soon, I'm feeling a bit ill and wheezy, with all the mould and rust.

BEN: Okay. It's starting raining now anyway.

🌢🌢 🌢 🌢 🌢 🌢🌢

7.26 p.m.

BEN: What's this you're watching – looks very posh?!

ME: *Homes Of The Rich And Famous.* It's a resort on Long Island, New York, called the Hamptons. The mansions are owned by celebs like Steven Spielberg and Beyoncé. Some are worth twenty million. Look at the mega luxury, cutting edge design and enormous swimming pools. The richest live close to the beach front, and some of the mansions there are worth seventy-five million!

BEN: But you're not the slightest bit envious (laughing).

ME: Not one teeny, tiny bit! My mini, modest beach hut will be my little mansion (smiling widely).

BEN: And it's situated on a part of the coast called Hampton.

ME: Really?

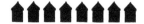

BEN: Here you are (handing me the A to Z open at the page showing the Kent coastline).

ME: Oh yes! Hampton. It should be called Little Kentish Hamptons. Then over time as the centuries fly by, it'll come to be known as Littletons.

BEN: Or Little Kentons.

ME: I could write a book about pixie creatures called the Little Kentons.

BEN: Or Herne Hutters.

ME: Yes. The Herne Hutters, who hibernate in the summer in secret caves that you can only explore if you have a hut, through a door in the floorboards. Only hut owners know about them and are sworn to secrecy. If they keep the secret they will be rewarded.

BEN: What is the reward?

ME: The pixies will give them magical potions to heal any ailment, physical or mental, bottled in tiny, sea-blue or seaweed-green glass bottles. These are crafted in the shape of seashells, seahorses and mermaids by the pixies in their caves. When the hut owners close up after the summer, the pixies appear to see if a request for a potion has been left for them. If you leave them a gift of shell-shaped chocolates, or an organic cream to soothe skin, made in Ireland from hand harvested seaweed, they will make your potion jar out a healing crystal, like blue lace agate – banded with pale blue wavy lines of many shades, it's a cooling, calming crystal with a soft energy, that brings peace of mind. They also love aquamarine – a green-blue crystal that reduces stress and was carried by sailors as a talisman against drowning.

BEN: What happens if the hut owners don't keep the pixie world a secret?

ME: The door to the pixie world in that particular hut is closed forever.

BEN: You intend to visit your hut when everyone else has closed up, after the summer. You could be the witch in your book who is there to greet the pixies when they emerge into hut land in the autumn. And have a meet'n'greet with a tasty buffet, served using doll's plates and cups.

ME: And share my knowledge of healing spells, and they could share their pixie knowledge with me.

BEN: I can see you painting a little door on the floor, in the corner of your hut.

ME: Or you could make one.

BEN: You and your imagination!

ME: Looking on the map, I can imagine roughly where my hut is.

BEN: You'll be tempted to sketch little beach huts with bunting on the A to Z.

ME: Possibly (smiling).

BEN: And a passing seagull?

ME: Maybe!

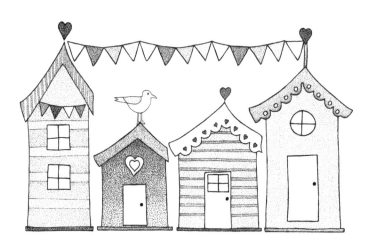

July

Tuesday 5th

1.00 p.m. I stand for a moment on a grassy hilltop, admiring the sun shining down on the row of brightly coloured beach huts, as pleasing to the eye as an array of radiant, rainbow coloured sweets in jars. The red and white, stripy huts – humbugs. The lime green huts – chocolate limes. Yellow huts – sherbet lemons. Pink – strawberry bonbons. The beautiful, blue and yellow hut is the sweet of my choice.

1.05 p.m. A wonderfully cool, gentle breeze blows my fine, wispy hair across my face. I brush it away from my eyes as I look up to admire my newly painted hut, stroking the silky, blue and yellow paintwork like I'm stroking the coat of a beloved cat.

ME: You and Bill have done a smashing job, *thank you so much!*

BEN: We're Bill and Ben, your beach hut men. Do you like the blue?

ME: No. *I absolutely love it!!*

BEN: What about the banisters?

ME: The bright, lemony yellow is lovely too. An improvement on the dull white, and will match the sunshine design when it's repainted..... Oh, I see you mended the wobbly banister.

BEN: Yeah, Bill gave me a hand.

ME: I heard a joke on the radio. Why did the man with one hand cross the road?

BEN: Dunno, why did the man with one hand cross the road?

ME: To get to the second hand shop.

BEN: Very good (smiling).

ME: When the metal bits are black and shiny, the hut will look good as new.

BEN: We decided to keep nearly all the existing fittings, aside from the bolt catch that fell to bits. The other parts will be okay, now we've wire-brushed them, and the Hammerite paint will stabilize the metal.

ME: Sounds good.

BEN: We were thinking, the decking and lower deck step looks a bit scruffy now. We could paint some floor paint on them.

ME: I'd like that. They seem dull and there's a lot of paint spots on them now. I notice other hutters leave their decking scruffy, but I think painted will look nice. It'll be all hands on deck.

BEN: Yeah!

ME: Oh, another joke I heard on the radio. A man was bemused when he bought a dog from a blacksmith. He'd only just brought it home and it had already made a bolt for the door.

BEN: Another good one! When Bill and I were last down here we met the neighbours on our right. Jane and Tom. Nice elderly couple. They had a friendly little dog.

ME: Lovely. What breed?

BEN: Dunno, some sort of – I dunno.

ME: Never mind (giggling). Lets have a look inside the hut.

ME: Ooh, seems a lot bigger without the clutter. And smells a lot better now you've removed so much stuff. The little blue, wooden table, will look nice when it's repainted.

BEN: Thought you'd like to keep the wooden ladder too.

ME: Yes, could come in useful and will look good repainted white. And we can see the floor tiles now. They look very grubby!

BEN: Yeah, they must come up. There's another layer of dirty tiles underneath. And lino under that. Look.

ME: Ugh.

BEN: You could have cushioned vinyl flooring – I've seen a driftwood pattern online.

ME: Sounds perfect.

BEN: And the hut will smell even better with a new floor.

ME: Think I'll keep the curtain rail, and the curtain looks
            in good condition. I like the duck egg blue and soft,
            thick cotton material. It just needs a good wash with
            a scented fabric conditioner. I'll take it home today.

BEN: The hut number needs screwing back on, on the back
            of the hut. Would you like it painted yellow?

ME: Yes please. It'll be nice and clear for the postman to
            see.

BEN: You'd better have a letterbox then!

WE LAUGH

1.17 p.m.   While Ben plods off on his pebbly walk to the pier, I
            enjoy a peaceful perch on the decking, like a watchful
            birdie. There are only a couple of families a few huts
            away and I love the distant, fun, seaside sounds of
            laughter. I imagine a lot of hutters come down at the
            weekends. I'll enjoy spending time at the hut in the
            week, when there's not a lot of people about, and in
            autumn when the weather is chillier, because Bill
            and Ben, my beach hut men, are going to make me
            an inner door. Bill says it should have portholes for
            windows. Nice idea. I will have some sort of heat-
            ing installed too.

            After a beautiful long daydream, I potter in the hut
            and I notice there's a rusty, seagull wall hook and
            seaside themed wall art that I could repaint. Or, as
            Henry Cole says, on *Find it, Fix it, Flog it* – upcycle.

            There are quite a few china mugs in good condition.

I will take them home and give them a very hot wash. We have plenty of mugs, so I will give some to an animal charity and the rest I will keep at the hut. I like some of the designs – colourful beach huts, navy and white stripes, and a couple of Herne Bay Pier Trust mugs, with a black and white photo of the pier (taken before half of it collapsed into the sea) and the promenade. It looks, judging by the motorcars, like the photo was taken in the fifties, and appears a popular holiday destination.

I'll keep the couple of tea trays too, with bright, jolly seaside paintings of stripy deckchairs, buckets and spades and sandcastles. After a hot wash and removal of the mildew spots they should come up a treat and look good as new.

2.07 p.m.   I hear Ben crunching towards the hut after his pebbly plod to the café on the pier. He perches beside me on the decking.

BEN: Happy?

ME: Very.

Monday 11th

10.06 a.m.

ME: It's *far too hot!* I'm so glad you and Bill went to the hut yesterday before it got *this hot!*

BEN: So am I. The car boot is chocker.

ME: Chocolate?

BEN: *Chocker!*.... The boot is full up of bin bags, stuffed with grubby old floor tiles and lino, ready to take to the tip.

ME: It can't have been easy taking the floor up. Thank you *so much*. You and Bill must treat yourself to a tasty Indian meal on me, at the nice Indian restaurant we spotted on the promenade.

BEN: We will!

ME: What sort of state are the floorboards in?

BEN: They're okay. In good nick.

ME: That's a relief.

BEN: I've booked a slot for a dump trip tomorrow at three o'clock.

ME: Great.

BEN: When I was in Wilko earlier, I saw a very comfy looking recliner on sale, a really good bargain.

ME: Like my beach hut.

BEN: Yeah. It's padded, with stripy, seaside coloured material, and good for a person with ME who needs to recline a lot.

ME: Sounds wonderful!

BEN: I'll get one this afternoon before they all go.

ME: That'll be lovely.

BEN: When we next go down to the hut, you can have a look at all the stuff I got out of the cupboards and see if there's anything you want to keep or clean for a charity shop.

ME: Okay. I've already decided about the mugs and trays left on the worktop.

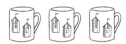

12.27 p.m.

ME: Do you know what's making that awful, really annoying loud noise outside our house? I don't want to close the windows, it's so hot!

BEN: There's a man sitting outside in his car. He's got a fan that switches on and off.

ME: Now I feel famous.

BEN: Why?

ME: There's an annoying fan outside that I wish would go away.

3.22 p.m.

ME: I read in Weekly wife, it can be good to eat spicy food in hot weather. Capsaicin, the chemical found in spicy food, stimulates heart receptors in your mouth, enhancing circulation and causing sweating, which cools the body down.

BEN: I look forward to an Indian meal with Bill!

ME: And it can be a good idea to fill a hot water bottle with ice water, and place it on the cooling points of your body. The best places are behind your knees, your ankles, wrists or elbows.

BEN: Right. I'm off to get the lounger.

ME: And maybe some hot, spicy veg to go with dinner?

BEN: Possibly (smiling) and maybe some chocolate.

ME: I've gone off chocolate.

BEN: Am I hearing right?

ME: Yes, you are. I'm watching *Holidaying With Jane McDonald: The Caribbean*. She's in Granada, and is visiting a place where they make chocolate bars.

BEN: Why has that put you off chocolate? Surely not the hot vats of creamy, aromatic chocolate?

ME: Oh, no. They look tasty, ready to pour into moulds. And the cocoa trees are lovely, with big pods – fifty beans a pod! They are dried in huge trays called bean beds, outside in the sunshine.

BEN: Sounds good.

ME: Yes.

BEN: I hear a big *but* coming on.

ME: It was the brown, wrinkly old lady, with wrinkly, grubby looking bare feet, that put me off choc, as she shuffled around in a bean bed, so the beans would be evenly dried. Bless her heart.

BEN: Ah. But no doubt you'll get over it in half an hour.

ME: Yes (grinning). The spice market that Jane visited looked good though. Enticing. Wonderful, vibrant, spicy reds, yellows and browns. I could verily smell the amazing aromas filling the air. Scents to make your nostrils, taste buds and eyebrows dance with excitement, all at once. You'd love it there.

BEN: I really fancy a spicy dinner now........ I'm off into town. When I'm in Sainsbury's I'll get something spicy, and a bar of chocolate may fall into my basket.

ME: Chocolate and spice and something else nice.

BEN: I hear some verse coming on.

ME: *Chocolate and spice*
And something else nice
At a verily, lovely
Affordable price

Thursday 14th

11.32 a.m.

BEN: Parcel for you.

ME: Oh, I wonder what it is.

BEN: I expect it's your Hammerite.

ME: Hematite? I haven't ordered any crystals.

BEN: Your white *Hammerite* paint. For the rusty, decorative, wall hooks and wall art you're going to repaint, or as you say, upcycle.

ME: Ah yes. White paint. Not black crystal.

ME: It says on the tin, there's no need for primer or undercoat. I've already given the metalwork a brush and clean, so just one coat needed. I found old Halloween paper cups under the sink, to use when I need to clean my brush with thinners. They have a sweet, bat design. Look.

BEN: Very nice dear. Very batty. Like you.

ME: Thanks (smiling).

ME: My vinyl, driftwood flooring sample arrived while you were out. So things are drifting along nicely. I love the design.

BEN: It'll feel soft under bare feet.

ME: And non-slippery, so our beach hut neighbour's dog can visit and scamper around, and not slip on its paws. Best of all, it will be low maintenance – two words I'm very fond of.

BEN: Me too (yawning).

2.02 p.m.

ME: I've found my hematite crystal.

BEN: Didn't know you were looking for it.

ME: I wasn't until you mentioned the Hammerite, that I thought of it. An interesting crystal, it's effective at grounding and protecting. It harmonizes the mind, body, and spirit. And –

BEN: Is that the time?.... I'm off to meet Les for a coffee in town. Then I'll get some tester pots for the hut.

4.00 p.m.

ME: Hope you enjoyed a good catch-up with Les.

BEN: Yeah. It was great to see him.

ME: How did the shopping for beach hut go?

BEN: I got a floor mop and bleach to clean the floorboards. Homebase didn't have a tester pot for the blue you liked, but I got four from Wilko – the ones I showed you on the internet that we both liked. Here you are.

ME: They look different from what you showed me online. Two of them are nice..... I can't wait till the inside of the hut is painted and the beautiful driftwood flooring is down.

BEN: I like the Surf Blue.

ME: Yes, so do I. But it looks more like a summer's day sky blue to me. The moody blue looks a bit dull and –

BEN: Moody?

ME: Yes. It's a sort of pale, duck egg blue. Cloudless looks a sort of grey cloud colour. Summer Blue has a touch of lilac. I like it. Do you?

BEN: Yeah.

ME: It's very hard to tell what the colour will be like though, on a wall, when you're looking at a little pot.

BEN: I'll paint all four pots on the hut wall, so you can make a decision.

ME: That would be *luverlee* (grinning from ear to ear).

BEN: We're in for very hot weather at the weekend and into the next week, so I'll pop down to the hut and give it a good clean tomorrow – bleach the walls and floor to get rid of mould and mildew. It should dry quickly in this weather, so I'll be able to paint the tester pots on the walls for madam to view.

ME: Sounds good! And yes, I heard on the radio we're going to have record breaking temperatures and there've been *extreme hot weather* warnings. Monday is going to be the hottest day on record in Britain – or maybe it's Tuesday.

BEN: Or both days.

ME: I feel a little faint just thinking about it.

ME: The lighthouse and sailing boat wall art and wall hooks that I'm painting white, will look good on a Surf Blue or Summer Blue wall.

BEN: Yeah.

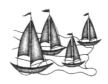

ME: So will the mirror with the frame painted white. And I could have a shelf painted –

BEN: White (grinning).

ME: I'm thinking a wooden mug tree would be nice for some of the mugs that were left in the hut. And a wooden kitchen roll holder would be good too. I could paint both –

BEN: White?

ME: Yes (grinning). And I do love kitchen roll. I wonder if you can still get the beach hut and bunting design. That used to be one of my favourite designs.

BEN: Now there's a surprise.

ME: Do you remember me writing poetry on pieces of roll?

BEN: I do!

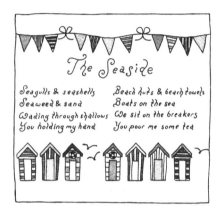

5.00 p.m.   We're in the kitchen. Ben is making a cuppa and I'm placing cans of food for the cats and foxes on a shelf.

ME: A shelf on one of the walls in my hut would help to make it look cosy. I could put spell books, sketch pads, notepads and seaside ornaments on it.

BEN: Artily placed.

ME: Yes (giggling). One of the mugs left in the hut has blue and white stripes. It will look good with my pens and pencils in it.

BEN: Paint brushes too, in case you fancy doing a spot of watercolour painting?

ME: Spot is the right word when it starts to spit with rain, when you are painting outdoors with watercolour and little spots of rain start to tap here and there on your artwork. I quite like the effect.

BEN: Improves your work.

WE LAUGH

ME: I'd like a clock for the hut.

BEN: I'll have a look online.

ME: And I'm thinking, if you can get some hooks, I could hang my battery operated hurricane lamp from the rafters. And the coloured glass balls in the thick string that I washed, have cleaned-up nicely.

BEN: Maybe some fish netting with shells and starfish?

ME: I don't think I'll go that far! Although I may bring some of my shell collection.

Monday 25th

10.05 a.m.

BEN: I have driftwood delights for you.

ME: Ooh, chocolates that look like driftwood?

BEN: Er, no.

ME: Driftwood chocolates sound nice though. Like those shell-shaped chocolates I love, that have the nutty filling. Can't recall what they're called..... the nutty filling was invented by a famous person's chef who boiled nuts in, erm.....

BEN: Driftwood?

ME: Sugar!

BEN: The driftwood flooring and clock to match have arrived. I'll open up the roll of flooring so you can see it, and get the clock out of the packaging – it's *very* well wrapped.

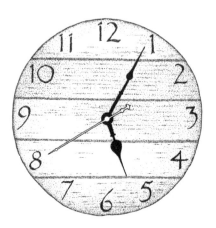

ME: I love them both! The flooring looks like *real* driftwood, and feels nicely spongy and soft. The driftwood design clock is *really nice* too. I like the tinted shades of blue in places, and sweet, delicate clock hands. I think it will look good above the mirror on the back wall of the hut.

BEN: I've painted the mirror frame white.

ME: I'll look forward to seeing that, and take the clock when we go to the hut today.

BEN: And I've painted the four tester pots on the wall so madam can have a peruse and choose.

10.36 a.m. We are off to beach hut city. Weather is perfect.

Warm. Not too hot. Pleasant breeze. There's some rain expected later in the Herne Bay area, but that will not be a problem, with a wee roof over our heads.

11.28 a.m.   The tide is in and it feels lovely to be out. Lovely to be back, welcomed with open arms by a warm sea breeze. The huts standing side by side as if hugging each other.

I embrace the beautiful day.

There's hardly anyone about. An elderly couple walk their little white dog. Two black headed seagulls bob happily, side by side on the undulating waves. A man waves to a young blonde woman, who runs towards him. They cuddle and laugh a lot.

Lovely.

11.31 a.m.

BEN: Bill has done a very good job, painting the sun on the roof.

ME: Oh, yes. It looks *fabulous!* Radiant yellow on a summer blue sky! I'll write and thank him, and send him a *big* thank you. First I'll give my hut a big hug.

BEN: You used to be a tree hugger. Now you're a hut hugger (laughing)……. Time to open up.

ME: You remembered to write the names of the tester pot colours next to the patches! I'm impressed (perusing the patches of blue on the wall, like an artist admiring paintings at the Tate Gallery, head on one side).

BEN: They look good.

ME: Too good. I *love* them all. The blues look so much better than I imagined when I saw the pots. I want to use them all.

BEN: I thought you'd say that.

ME: Using all four could get expensive, so I think the surf blue for the back wall. It will look good surrounding the white-framed mirror, reflecting the sky and sea. And I'm thinking, Summer Blue for the other walls. The little wooden table could be Surf Blue too. I'm tempted to paint the ceiling Cloudless Blue but I think it looks okay as it is.

BEN: Yeah.

11.41 a.m.   We sit on the decking enjoying the sea breeze and relaxing sound of the waves.

ME: *I bought some little tester pots*
Different shades of blue
I can't decide which one to use
I may use every hue

BEN: *She bought a little beach hut*
She painted every hue
This made her very happy
And made me happy too

WE LAUGH

11.52 a.m.	Back in the hut.

BEN: Bill and I thought the floorboard, just inside the door is getting a bit springy.

ME: Ah, I see what you mean. Can it be sorted?

BEN: We thought the best thing to do, is fit a very thin metal plate across it. I found just the thing on the internet, shall I order it?

ME: Yes please.

BEN: It will be invisible when your driftwood flooring is down.

ME: I'm looking forward to that! I thought at first, I could have just cleaned floorboards, but they look stained and, well, not very nice at all really.

12.35 p.m.

ME: Hungry?

BEN: Very.

ME: Time for crisps sandwiches then.

BEN: If you do spell work here, will you be a sand witch?

ME: I will (cackling quietly, so as not to frighten the neighbours).

ME: I so love it that Bill has done such a great job painting the sun. If Jerry saw it, his heart would smile.

BEN: Yeah.

ME: The decking will look good painted a sort of sea-weedy green, if you know what I mean.

BEN: Yes dear.

ME: I wonder if the famous artist Tracey Emin from Margate, got excited about painting her beach hut in Whitstable.

BEN: She had a hut in Whitstable, did she?

ME: Yes. I read about her in an old copy of Marie Clare mag the other day. At one time she went to the same art college as me.

BEN: Did you meet her?

ME: No, but that would have been interesting, she's quite a character. I don't think she was there long, and ended up going to the Maidstone College Of Art, at around the time I was renting a room very near there.

BEN: You might have passed her on the Tonbridge road.

ME: Yes. These days I like to play spot the art student, when you take me to an appointment at the hospital or dentist.

BEN: I remember last time, the girl with green and blue hair and red and yellow stripy tights caught your eye.

>July

ME: And a very tall man with long, wild, black hair, wearing a multi-coloured jumper, singing to himself looked eccentric and arty.

BEN: I remember!

ME: Tracey Emin had her beach hut installed in an art gallery – the White Cube.

BEN: Was her hut painted white?

ME: That was the name of the gallery. From the tiny photo in the mag, her hut looks a dull, miserable blue and yellow.

BEN: Unlike yours – a happy blue and yellow.

ME: Yes... She sold hers in the year two thousand. It was entitled, *The Last Thing I Said To You Was Don't Leave Me Here.*

BEN: Sad.

ME: Yes. But the price she sold it for wasn't sad! Charles Saachi bought it for seventy-five thousand pounds. It was probably worth around ten thousand pounds at the time.

BEN: Blimey.

ME: Crazy art world eh!

BEN: Mad.

ME: I remember strolling past the beach huts in Whitstable back in the nineties, admiring them and dreaming wistfully that I would own one, one day.

BEN: Whitstable-fully.

ME: Yes. I may have admired Tracey's hut at one time... If Charles Saachi reinstalled her hut on the beach at Whitstable now, it may be worth a small fortune!

BEN: Yeah.

ME: I wonder if he's installed the hut at the end of his garden – a conversation piece for his summer garden parties and the place where drinks are served. Especially drinks that Tracey loves.

BEN: What does she love?

ME: In the article, she said she used to have a handbag that held four beers, half a bottle of brandy and cigarettes. But eventually gave up spirits and cigarettes. She enjoys wine now.

BEN: So there could be a tribute corner in the hut with her fave wine, brandy and cigarettes.

ME: And pictures of cats.

BEN: Is she a cat lover?

ME: I don't know. But when she was speaking in public and a bit drunk –

BEN: Not surprising, if she carried beer and brandy around with her.

ME: Yes (giggling). She would make cat meow noises during her speeches.

BEN: Diamanda and Lovely may have understood what she was saying.

ME: Or be bemused.

BEN: Be-meowsed.

ME: If she's a cat lover, I approve. Though I've never seen cats as the subject of her artwork.

BEN: When you're a famous writer and illustrator, will you install your beach hut in a gallery for sale?

ME: Never.

BEN: You'll never sell your hut or never be famous?

ME: Both (giggling). It will be passed down to my little, witchy niece, who always loved to build sand-castles and collect shells, beside the seaside. And now she's a bigger witch, loves to perform spells using shells, potions, sandcastles and the power of the sea. Of all water magic, that which flows from the sea is the most potent.

BEN: I hear some verse coming on.

ME: *Shells, spells and sandcastles*
The power of the sea

BEN: *It all works well together*

ME: *With love from you to me!*

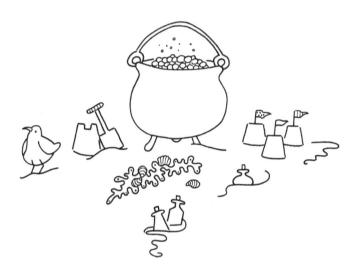

Chapter Four

August

Saturday 6th

ME: I feel a little nervous about going to the hut today.

BEN: Why's that?

ME: It sounds a bit silly, but I had this *very* vivid dream that when we got to the beach hut, we found the tide had come in *so far* that the hut was flooded. The floor was under almost a foot of water, with black seaweed floating on the surface.

BEN: Does the thought of the hut flooding worry you?

ME: No. But I recall listening to the radio before I nodded off to sleep, and heard a man talking about climate change and rising sea levels.

BEN: Ah.

ME: The dream continued with us wading through the water and hearing screams in the distance. Then we watched in horror as the pier cracked and crumbled, eventually crashing into the sea.

BEN: I expect you heard on the radio that the heatwave has made some houses crack – especially in our part of the country.

ME: Yes!

BEN: Camomile tea dear?

ME: Please.

11.38 a.m.   We arrive in Herne Bay and park on the roadside at the top of the hill, almost opposite my hut.

ME: Looks like the tide is going out.

BEN: No flooding then!

ME: And the pier looks fine (giggling).

11.47 a.m.

ME: I can't help admiring again, the smashing job Bill has done of painting the lemony yellow sun. It radiates so beautifully out of the blue, making the once sad hut, bright and happy. And the metal bits you've painted with black gloss, look great. Well done you!

BEN: Think I did a good job (smiling).

ME: Can't wait to see inside now.

11.49 a.m.

ME: What a *beautiful* soft blue (stroking the wall). I like the matt finish, and the Surf Blue on the back wall looks *really* nice behind the white framed mirror.

BEN: The Summer Blue looks fresh and clean.

ME: And no more musty, rusty smells.

BEN: I'll put the white shelf up next. The white hook and wall art you painted will look good on the Summer Blue.

ME: I've brought my tailor's chalk, to mark where I'd like the shelf and hook – shelf and hooks for my ornaments and books.

BEN: Do you feel some verse coming on?

ME: No, not at the moment. But I'm feeling inspired. A little light bulb is shining brightly with excitement, in the interior design part of my brain.

BEN: I can see a sparkle in your eye.

ME: I don't like the driftwood flooring though.

BEN: Oh (looking crestfallen).

ME: *I love, love it!*

BEN: Brother Dave did a good job didn't he.

ME: A most *grand job!* Did he have special cutters?

BEN: No, just a Stanley knife. I got a pack of new blades.

ME: Is it stuck down?

BEN: I just stuck the edges with a little PVA adhesive.

ME: I'll take my flatties off so I can feel what it's like with bare feet...... soft.... cool.... clean.

BEN: Your toes are dancing.

ME: I've happy feet.

         Oh! They do like to beside the seaside
         Oh! They do like to be beside the sea

11.59 a.m.   We sit in contented silence on the decking, just watching the waves rolling as the tide gently ripples out. Bathers wave to their roly-poly family on the beach, who are bringing food out of their hut – lots of plates of sandwiches and tasty things in pastry, for a fabulous picnic.

ME: Another heatwave is on the way. Summer rolls on.

BEN: Fancy a large veggie sausage roll?

ME: Not half.

12.04 p.m.

ME: I'm not looking forward to another heatwave. But I had to giggle, when I heard a presenter on Radio Kent say he had family visiting from Australia. They weren't very happy with our baking hot weather. They said they couldn't wait to go home, back to Australia, because the British weather was too hot for them. That's something I've never heard before!

BEN: Yeah (laughing). I expect there will be hose pipe bans.

ME: *Hose pipe bans*
And making plans
For days beside the sea

It's nice to sit
Just watching waves
Just us

BEN: *Just you and me*

ME: My stars with Cosmic Colin, say that going with the flow comes naturally to me. So I might have a little paddle in the shallows.

BEN: Did you bring a towel?

ME: Ah, no. I'll remember next time.

1.00 p.m. It starts to sprinkle with rain, so we set up our festival chairs in the shelter of the hut, and sit comfortably.

BEN: What are you up to?

ME: Tying string to the handle of my hurricane lamp, so I can hang it from the rafters when you put some hooks up.

BEN: I'll give the rafters a coat of Danish oil.

ME: That'll be lovely. On the upcycling programme I watch, they recommend you wear gloves when using Danish oil. And I notice they've been using a lot of blues. Light blues to brighten old, wooden, chairs and tables or whatever. The other day they used, what looked like the same blue as my hut. Apparently blue is on trend at the moment. I've never been on trend in my life!

BEN: Neither have I.

ME: What is blue and not heavy?

BEN: Dunno, what is blue and not heavy?

ME: Light blue.

ME: I heard something on Heart Radio that made my heart smile – made me feel very fortunate to have my own beach hut.

BEN: What was that?

ME: A young man was talking about how much he loved walking on the North Norfolk coast. I don't know if the interview was about beach huts, I only heard the tail end of it, but he talked about how much he loved the beach huts along the coast, and said there was no way he could afford one. So he built one in his back garden and would love to sit, just watching the rain and listen to raindrops falling on the roof.

I remember once sitting on the breakers on Whitstable beach, watching very dramatic storm clouds rolling from the horizon towards the beach. I enjoyed the speckle of raindrops, as the clouds approached, until big, fat raindrops fell on my face. I didn't want to go home, but had no umbrella or raincoat. Which didn't bother me much but the person I was with –

BEN: Didn't love rain clouds and rain as much as you.

ME: Do you remember that programme I heard on the radio about cloud formations a little while ago? I told you about cirrus clouds.

BEN: Yeah.

ME: I didn't tell you about my favourite clouds, cumulonimbus. The name is from the Latin cumulus – heaped, and nimbus – rainstorm.

BEN: That's what inspired the name of one of the broomstick's in J K Rowling's Harry Potter books then – the Nimbus Two Thousand.

ME: Yes!... When these clouds occur as a thunderstorm, they can be referred to as thunderheads.

BEN: Good name.

ME: And a name for big, gruff men in a bad temper.

BEN: Yeah (laughing).

ME: Back to my Whitstable memory. The clouds rolling towards the beach were dark purple and evil yellow. I called them bruisers because –

BEN: They looked like a bruise.

ME: They did. A huge, painful bruise. The gods showing their wrath – how pained they are feeling for the way we are treating our beautiful planet. I didn't want to go home, just feel their tears on my face.

BEN: You must have been having a bad day dear. It's raining now, so you can sit and watch raindrops in the shelter of your hut. Or venture outside and do a little witchy dance on the beach, to say sorry to the gods of our beautiful planet.

ME: I think for now I'll just sit, watching the rain, send out good thoughts and enjoy our sandwiches.

BEN: Without them getting soggy.

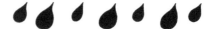

ME: I feel a Julie Andrews coming on:

           Raindrops on pebbles
           They sparkle and glisten
           The call of the seagulls
           We just sit and listen
           Hanging my lantern
           With a piece of string

BEN: *These are a few of your*
           Favourite things

ME: One of your favourite things is eating.

BEN: Yep (tucking into a third sandwich).

ME: *He said to her*
           It's just a shed by the sea
           And she said to him
           But it fills my heart with glee

BEN: *Then he said to her*
           Would you like some tea

ME: *And she replied*

BEN: *Most certainly*

ME: I can't get the lid off this flask.

She said to him
Can't get the lid off this flask

BEN: *And he said to her*
         You only have to ask

Tuesday 16th

9.42 a.m.

BEN: *Ow! Ouch!*

ME: What have you done?

BEN: Stubbed me toe.

ME: I just heard a joke on the radio – My wife told me to stop acting like a flamingo. So I put my foot down.

BEN: Thank you. That makes me feel a *whole lot* better.

ME: I feel a *whole lot* better, now it's cooler and there's a gentle tapping on the window – the rain is here at last.

BEN: Yeah, at long last, after far too many days of heat.

ME: I can almost hear the garden sighing with relief, now its thirst has been quenched. And the straw-coloured lawn opposite our house will come back to life again.

BEN: We'll sleep better too.

ME: Yes (yawning). And we can close the windows. The young foxes were making such a din in the early hours, they kept waking me up. When I did get some sleep, I had *such surreal* dreams about the beach hut.

BEN: What's new! Flooding?... Crumbling pier?.. Sharks? ... Mermaids?

ME: Funny you should say that. There was a shark in the dream. Probably because I heard a joke on the radio, on the Paul Miller show. A crocodile, a shark and a giant spider walk into a bar. There's no punchline. It's just a typical night in Australia.

BEN: So there was a crocodile, shark and giant spider in your dream?

ME: Yes (giggling). Also young, seaweed-green foxes, barking, splashing about and dancing in the shallows with turquoise fishes, golden lobsters and mermaids with silvery tails, singing.

BEN: An average night for you then.

ME: I'm looking forward to when we get the storms.... I read a quote I liked in a gift catalogue yesterday, by Vivian Green:

Life isn't about waiting
for the storm to pass...
It's about learning to dance in the rain

BEN: Good quote.

ME: And there's a quote I like by Jack Handey:

If a kid asks where rain comes from,
I think a cute thing to tell him is,
God is crying.
And if he asks why God is crying,
another cute thing to tell him is,

Probably because of something you did.

BEN: Right, I'm off for my morning plod.

ME: Can you open this bottle of water please, before you go?

BEN: Yep.

ME: Would you mind hanging around for a little while. I've put a cat bed in the washing machine. The new, grey one. I haven't washed it before and I'm concerned that the washing machine may not like it, rattle about, flood the kitchen, or explode or something.

BEN: The machine should be fine. The cat bed doesn't weigh much, and it's squishy and springy. The thing the machine likes least is, for example, just a couple of towels and nothing else, because they soak up the water and sit, like small heavy lumps in one place. This makes the drum very off balance and the whole thing shakes around.

ME: You've just described me (giggling). I'm often like a wet towel. I soak up plenty of bottles of mineral water and sit like a heavy lump in one place, which can make me feel a little unbalanced. Then I wobble to the kitchen.

BEN: What are you like (laughing).

ME: A wet towel. A bit washed out.

BEN: When we next go to the hut, you'll be like a mermaid, washed-up on the shore. I'll carry you to your decking, where you can sit, flap your tail fin happily, sun yourself and comb your long hair, like in Mr Waterhouse's famous painting.

WE LAUGH

BEN: I expect you're looking forward to your next trip to the hut.

ME: Very much so.

BEN: We could take your new sunlounger.

ME: Yes. It looks ever so comfy. Did you know sunloungers date back to the ancient Aztecs, who loved to sunbathe?

BEN: I don't expect their lounger was as comfy as yours.

ME: Probably made of scratchy reeds, twigs and leaves or something.

BEN: Yeah.

ME: I'll take the seaside ornaments I bought the other day in Rye, too.

BEN: They'll look good on the shelf I've painted white.

ME: They will!..... It was so enjoyable to have a drink at The Mermaid Inn in Rye, when we were shopping there. Brought back happy memories of the nights we've spent there celebrating our birthdays. And everyone was social distancing that day too.

BEN: Apart from the wasp.

ME: Yes!

BEN: I've painted the wooden mug tree white and the kitchen roll holder.

ME: Great. I'm looking forward to hanging my beach hut mugs on the mug tree and roll on the kitchen roll holder – a seaside design would be good.

BEN: That doesn't surprise me. And both are on a *beautifully clean* work surface.

ME: You know how to excite a girl.

BEN: And you should take the mermaid you bought.

ME: Oh, yes. The lovely little cast iron mermaid – a gorgeous, glowing seaweed-green with gold flecks. She'll look good on my decking, but will need to be cemented down in case someone tries to steal her away. You'll have to carry her down from the car to the hut, she's *far too heavy* to for me.

BEN: Certainly dear. Open things for you.... carry cats to the vet..... carry shopping..... carry rubbish out for the bin men..... carry heavy mermaids to the beach.

WE LAUGH

1.47 p.m.

BEN: Why the sad face?

ME: Wish I was at my hut. Or sipping a cool drink at The
            Mermaid Inn. The TV is so boring today.

BEN: Here's your copy of Celebrity Weekly. Keep you quiet
            – I mean wonderfully entertained.

ME: Thanks. I'll enjoy a good old nosey, celeb peruse......
            Jennifer Lopez and Ben Afflec look like they are
            putting on a wonderful romantic display. Jen's floral
            dress by Oscar de la Renta is very lovely don't you
            think – look.

BEN: Very nice. Very flowery.

ME: But not the large, shell-pink handbag, no doubt de-
            signer. Doesn't go with anything she's wearing.

BEN: I quite agree (yawning).

ME: They are on their honeymoon in Paris – pages of
            photos of them cuddling, taking selfies, laughing
            and holding hands.

BEN: Are you moved to write romantic poetry?

ME: Maybe a few lines.

            Laughing, cuddles and a selfie
            Jen's no-longer on the shelfie
            They like to own designer brands
            Enjoying Paris holding hands

BEN: It may not be long before you're reading about their bitter divorce.

ME: And who gets custody of the large, ugly, shell-pink designer handbag.

BEN: Yeah.

ME: The Beckhams seem to be having a fabulous time too, enjoying a lavish vacation on their five million pound super-yacht, off the coast of Italy – sunbathing, sipping cool drinks on deck, taking photos of each other and their children. David shows off his toned torso and Victoria, always thin, is even more so. Am I moved to poetry. I don't think so.

BEN: Orlando Bloom looks bloomin' ridiculous, posing on what looks like a tropical beach.

ME: I can't see what that young singer sees in him. Can't remember her name. My niece likes her. She sang about fireworks and tigers. Wonderful voice. *What is her name?*..... Brought out a perfume. The bottle in the shape of a cat, called *Purr* I think. I bought it for my my niece a few years ago.... She stars in an advert about, something to do with food..... Very colourful costume changes.

BEN: Haven't a clue who she is. Does it matter?

ME: No, not really. Kim Kardashian's little daughter and her cousin look sweet, dressed as mermaids with rainbow tails, don't they. They are on decking, somewhere exotic I imagine.

BEN: Very nice (yawning).

ME: This week's feel-good read in the book section looks intriguing. I especially like *The Lighthouse Bookshop* by Sharon Gosling – nice cover. The write-up is good, book sounds atmospheric and enchanting.

BEN: It caught your eye because it has a lighthouse on the cover and you've got seaside on the brain these days!

ME: It does sound like a perfect read for an afternoon beside the seaside.

BEN: Shall I order it for you?

ME: Yes please.

          No entertainment is so cheap as
          reading, any pleasure as lasting.

BEN: Who said that?

ME: Can't remember. Lady Mary something.

BEN: Good quote. You'll *love* this email that just arrived. Come and look.

          Hi Ben

          Hope you are both well and enjoying the hut during this long spell of sunny weather.

          I saw the hut today and love the colour scheme.

          Thanks so much for keeping the sunburst, it means a lot to us.

          All best Wishes

          Jerry

Friday 26th

9.00 a.m.

ME: What a perfect day for a trip to the seaside. Sunshine and a cool breeze. I wonder if we'll see a shark?

BEN: Been dreaming again about sharks and crocodiles, green foxes, blue fishes and mermaids with silvery tails again, have we?

ME: No. I heard on Radio Kent this morning that a basking shark has just been spotted swimming off our coast. People are being advised not to swim in the sea.

BEN: Where?

ME: Folkestone.

BEN: I expect you'd like to drive down there, just to spot a nice shark fin swimming about.

ME: That would be fun. I expect quite a few people will just happen to be visiting there! But Herne Bay will suit me fine today.

BEN: It'll be the grand inaugural boil, using your new kettle and miniature stove.

ME: Yes! My cute little whistling kettle – I like the silver, curvy design, with a black handle and knob to match on the lid. Like a silver, iced cake with a black cherry on top.

BEN: When we get to the beach and you plod off to the toilets, I can greet you on your return, as you step onto the decking, with the whistling kettle. Like sailors with their pipes when they welcome an officer or important person onto a ship.

ME: Will you salute me?

BEN: Of course!

11.27 a.m. The kettle is whistling merrily as I step onto the deck of my ship and Ben salutes me with a sailor's twinkle in his eye.

BEN: Welcome aboard madam. Cuppa?

ME: Decaf coffee with a dash of rum – just joking.

BEN: Any preference of mug milady. Beach huts? Blue and white stripes? Herne Bay pier?

ME: The one with the black and white photo of fifties Herne Bay, please. I was watching a programme I enjoyed in the seventies, the other day, *Upstairs Downstairs*. Do you remember? The grumpy cook, Mrs Bridges? Ruby and Rose and the other servants downstairs?

BEN: Yeah, and Mr Hudson.

ME: Upstairs, there was Richard and James. I can't re-member her Ladyship's name. Oh, and there was, their daughter, what *was* her name?

BEN: Georgie?

ME: Georgiana!....... Hudson reminds me of Carson, in *Downton Abbey*.

BEN: Yeah.

ME: Anyway, Mrs Bridges was looking through a photo album of seaside holidays they'd enjoyed in Herne Bay. The series was set in the early nineteen hundreds so I wonder if it was a popular seaside resort then.

BEN: Do you require biscuits with your coffee milady (Hudson voice).

ME: That would be lovely thank you Hudson (Her Ladyship voice). I must say this lounger is most agreeable. Who needs a Beckham super-yatch when you have –

BEN: A super-stripy lounger, a super mug of coffee and your favourite biscuits served up to you, after being whistled and saluted on the deck of your own ship, I mean beach hut, with a super-seaside view.

11.33 a.m. As we dunk our biscuits in coffee, we enjoy watching three little boys dunking each other in the shallows, shrieking with laughter.

ME: I have another quote for you I've just thought of, by Wallace Stevens.

BEN: *Wallace & Gromit: A Grand Day Out* is on tonight.

ME: Oh good. It's very funny when Wallace is distraught, because his cheese supply has run out, so he builds a spaceship with his dog, to fly to the moon because it's made of cheese. The animation and sound affects are brilliant. Remember the sound of Gromit sawing the wood? And the paint cans rattling in the cellar as the spaceship takes off, just like ours did when the housing estate was built opposite us?

BEN: Yeah.

ME: It will make you crave cheese and crackers though, and we don't have any in.

BEN: I'll pick up some from Sainsbury's on our way home.

ME: That'll be nice. What was I saying?

BEN: You were going to quote Wallace somebody.

ME: Oh yes. The little boys playing in the shallows made me think of it.

Most people read poetry, listening for echoes because the echoes are familiar to them. They wade through it the way a boy wades through water, feeling with his toes for the bottom: the echoes are the bottom.

BEN: Talking of bottoms, mine's a bit numb. I'll be off for a plod. Stretch me legs along beach hut city.

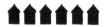

ME: The driftwood clock will look just right above the mirror.

BEN: Yeah, mark where you want me to hang it.

ME: I'm relieved it hasn't got a loud tick-tock, it would make me feel too sleepy because I sleep to a tick-tock sound.

BEN: The white shelf will look good too, on the blue wall. I see you didn't bring your seaside ornaments.

ME: Well, the summer is nearly over, and it will soon be closing-up-hut time for the winter, because I haven't got my inner doors or heating yet. Ornaments and books will only get dusty and damp.

BEN: I've just been chatting to the chap painting the old black hut near the loos. He's using a deep blue from B&Q – an exterior paint called Royal Blue. I thought it might be good for your decking.

ME: Sounds nice. Although I was thinking more a seaweed-green, if that's available.

BEN: I'll find out.

ME: *A royal blue*
        From B&Q
        Or a seaweed-green
        If you know what I mean

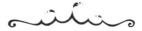

BEN: Are you enjoying *The Lighthouse Bookshop*?

ME: I've only read a few pages, but it's good so far. The story draws you in.

BEN: You've been very restrained. You got the book over a week ago but managed to save it for reading at the hut, because you do like to read beside the seaside.

ME: That I do. It's been like a box of chocolates calling out for me to leisurely indulge, choc after choc. Words have been calling out to me –

BEN: To leisurely indulge, page after page. I'll bet you couldn't resist just a little nibble of a paragraph or two?

ME: I did lift the lid for a quick glance, and a little bit of a read, here and there.

BEN: And a nice sniff between the pages, for the new book smell.

ME: I may have.

BEN: Like you love to inhale the sweet, minty aroma, when you open a box of After Eight mints.

ME: It was *so tempting* to curl up with the cats and a cuppa, and get completely lost in the story. And I do love where the story is set.

BEN: Where?

ME: Beautiful Scotland. I can so imagine being there.

BEN: The boat trip we took down Loch Ness was great.

ME: Yes. And the castle ruins that the boat stopped at were lovely. The loch was much bigger than I thought it would be, and we really enjoyed the trip. But it was a pity the monster, Nessie, was hiding that day, or having an afternoon nap.

BEN: The families of wild seals near Inverness made up for it.

ME: And the geese flying in V shapes, joining together to make an enormous wobbly V. I'd never seen anything like it! It's so much better to see these wonders in real life, instead of on a wildlife programme. And I'd never seen a massive sea eagle before. Do you remember when we were parked near a cliff edge, and it appeared, rising up from the sea and flew quite close, over our car.

BEN: Its wing span must have been as wide as the car.

ME: I looked up through the open sunroof, and it certainly filled that.

BEN: How did you know it was a sea eagle?

ME: We stopped at a little shop nearby with a notice in the window showing the eagle, and asking anyone who had spotted it, to let them know.

BEN: Did we?

ME: The shop was shut. Shame, I wanted to tell them, I was quite excited. Remember the swans?

BEN: Nope.

ME: It was early, one misty morning. We saw a flock of them flying quite low over a deserted sandy beach, near the water's edge. It was magical.

BEN: Oh, yeah.

ME: Like the geese.

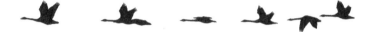

ME: My new book, *The Lighthouse Bookshop* arrived the day after you ordered it from Amazon, which brings to mind a joke I heard the other day. If you want to get pregnant in the Amazon, you get next day delivery.

BEN: I expect a lot of women going through pregnancy would like that!

12.32 p.m.   Ben crunches off along the pebbles for his morning exercise. I happily sit and listen to the crunching sound fade into the distance.

              The sound of rippling waves, calling seagulls, and a family laughing outside their beach hut in the distance, is so relaxing. I hear myself sigh deeply, and think to myself – this is nice. Then I return to Scotland and *The Lighthouse Bookshop*. Turning the page, I am soon engrossed and I smile to myself. I like it that there is a resident cat at the lighthouse.

              The cat had come with the lighthouse, but Rachel had no illusions he was hers. Eustace belonged to Cullen MacDonald, just as the tower did and always would, no matter that he no longer actually lived within its walls.

1.16 p.m.   Ben returns from his plod.

BEN: Time for sandwiches.

ME: Your wish is my command.

BEN: Still enjoying the book?

ME: Yes. And I can tell the author has a cat. She mentions things that only a cat lover would observe or consider. I've just started chapter seven.

BEN: Already?

ME: They're short chapters and easy to read. Lots of interesting characters, and they are *so well* described, I can see them quite clearly. Like I'm watching a film.

BEN: Maybe it *will* be made into a film.

ME: I wouldn't be surprised.

BEN: We'll have to wait and see (devouring an egg and cress sandwich).

ME: The cat in the lighthouse does what our Lovely does. I'll read you an extract:

           She went up into the kitchen and fed the cat, pausing for a moment to stroke him as he wolfed his food, feeling the purr reverberate through his familiar form.

BEN: That sounds just like Lovely, wolfing her food and purring at the same time (taking a huge bite out of another sandwich, then opening a bag of crisps and crunching away – crunch, crunch, crunch – the same rhythm as his plod on the pebbly beach, to the pier).

BEN: I'll get on with painting the ladder and small table.

ME: And I'll get back to Rachel and Eustace the cat at the lighthouse.

BEN: You'd better leave the book at the hut when we go home, or you'll finish it over the weekend.

ME: Good idea.

4.22 p.m. While Ben locks-up the hut, I pat shiny, blue wood and say goodbye. But not sadly. I don't feel blue, I feel sunshine yellow.

We slowly make our way up the winding path behind the huts to our car, parked at the top of the hill, patting a friendly little dog that stops to greet us, wagging its tail madly.

On reaching the car, I silently bid farewell to beach hut city. Land of the Herne hutters. I'm one of them now. No going back... I think I feel an Agatha Christie moment coming on.

5.44 p.m. We enjoy watching Wallace and Gromit making a spaceship, to fly to the moon made of cheese, for their grand day out – while we nibble cheese and crackers and look forward to *The Agatha Christie Hour* later, with dinner.

8.46 p.m.   Ben taps away on his laptop.

BEN: I've found a matt green for the decking, come and look.

ME: Hmm, deepest green looks nice.

BEN: It'll need to be varnished to make it weatherproof.

ME: Okay, that'll be good.

BEN: Or there's this colour.

ME: Quite a nice sort of teal. I read in Weekly Wife, it's the nation's favourite colour.

BEN: A greeny-blue.

ME: For people who like green and blue.

BEN: Like you.

ME: Teal is a nice colour, but I'm not sure I want it on my decking. Although I'd quite like a top in that shade.

BEN: You've got that look in your eye. I see some verse coming on.

ME: *I once knew a seal*
The colour of teal
He liked me to feed him
A tuna meal

His colour had
A certain appeal
And I said to him
Are you for real?

BEN: *And he replied*
           With an aquatic squeal

           Make up your mind woman!

ME: A seal would never say that. He'd say, yes, teal is very
           nice, but I think a deeper green would look better
           on your decking – go well with the blue and yellow
           of your beach hut. Then he'd give me his seal of
           approval smile, twitch his whiskers, and invite me
           to swim with him and the mermaids, who hang out
           under the pier.

BEN: Right. Deepest green it is.

ME: I heard a woman on the radio this morning say a
           wild, baby seal had come in through her cat flap and
           scared her cat. She heard the *slap, slap* sound of its
           flippers and thought, what on earth is that?!

BEN: Where does she live?

ME: I don't know, I only tuned in at the end of the inter-
           view. But she sounded Australian.

BEN: What happened to the seal?

ME: The woman rang a ranger person who came to collect
           it, and said it was common for seals to come inland
           at that time of year. But not into houses!

BEN: You'd love a seal to come in through our cat flap.

ME: That would be funny. The seal that swam into the river near us last year, who the marine saving people named Bradley, would have been most welcome to plod into our kitchen for a tuna snack and a bit of a gossip about what's going on in his watery world. I loved the photos you took of him to show me. He looked happy and well, but I'm glad he eventually returned safely to the sea.

BEN: He turned out to be a she.

ME: Oh yes!

BEN: Lovely and Diamanda would have growled at her if she'd come into the kitchen.

ME: The woman with the seal in her kitchen said the seal growled at her.

BEN: You would love a seal growling at you.

ME: That I would!... And a crocodile.

BEN: Do crocodiles growl?

ME: No idea. Maybe they do a scary grunt. Though they probably growl a lot when they have to go to the dentist.

BEN: I don't think a crocodile would fit in through our cat flap.

ME: I saw a video of this woman who liked crocodiles, on *Worlds Funniest Videos,* the other morning. The animal ones were good. The one I liked best, was the small crocodile appearing at this woman's kitchen door. She threw chicken pieces to it and it plodded into the kitchen to munch them with lots of big, shiny teeth.

BEN: It must have been to the dentist for a clean and polish. Was this in Australia?

ME: No idea, could have been. It looked quite a posh kitchen. Maybe it was in America, in Miami, near the Everglades.

BEN: A seal, a crocodile and a giant spider walk into a kitchen. There's no punchline, it's a typical day in Australia.

WE LAUGH

9.19 p.m. I curl up in bed, under the covers with a hot chocolate and a good book, looking forward to a good read – will Rachel uncover the truth?

BEN: Caught you! Secretly having an early night with *The Lighthouse Bookshop*. I thought you were going to leave it at the hut (laughing).

ME: Well, yes. I *was* going to. I *really intended* to. But I must have absent-mindedly slipped it into my bag.

September

Thursday 1st

8.37 a.m.

BEN: I see your nose is in the book again.

ME: It's a big book, so I still have lots, many more truly
        scrumptious pages to deliciously devour. And I'll save
        chapters to read for my next visit to the hut.

BEN: You're like our Lovely, wolfing her food down and
        purring at the same time.

ME: I'll try to pace myself with the mouth-watering
        mystery set on a Scottish coast, full of romance and
        intrigue. There's just been a dramatic fire in the story.

BEN: In the lighthouse?

ME: No. In the studio of one of the characters – an ec-
        centric artist who lives in the remote village near the
        lighthouse, and works by candlelight while she drinks
        wine.

BEN: Does she die?

ME: She's been rescued just in time. But things are not
        looking good for the lighthouse. It's future is uncert-
        ain, it could be knocked down. It's more a folly than
        a lighthouse, built by an eccentric landowner, just
        inland from the coast in Aberdeenshire. There's an
        eccentric writer and journalist too, who uncovers cor-
        ruption by people who want to knock the lighthouse
        down and build something.

BEN: Lots of eccentric characters then. I can see why you like the book dear. You'll have finished it by tomorrow.

ME: I'll try *really hard* to save the last few chapters for our next visit to the hut. It'll be fun reading about a lighthouse, with the sound of waves and seagulls in the background.

BEN: I can't see that happening. It'll be like you trying to leave the last crisp in the packet of your favourite cheese and onion crisps, or last chocolate digestive biscuit that must be eaten before it goes off.

ME: Or the last Malteser in the box. Rolling around. All alone. Enticing me. The sweet, brown sphere, wanting, waiting, eager to be crunched, like the pebbles at Herne Bay await happy, plodding feet. And the delightful centre longs to melt on the tongue, like warm waves melting into grains of sand.... You are right. I have no willpower.

WE LAUGH

9.27 a.m.   I switch the kettle on for a cuppa and the last biscuit in the packet. I'm in my bare feet, and as Ben enters the kitchen, I plod around the floor making a *slap, slap* sound near the cat flap.

BEN: What *are you doing?*

ME: I'm being a seal coming in through the cat flap. Remember? The woman in Australia who was talking on the radio, who had a young seal come in through her cat flap?

BEN: Oh, yeah (rolling eyes).

ME: Oh (groaning).

BEN: Are you making crocodile growling noises now?

ME: No, I've just trodden on something soft and wet. But I could attempt a crocodile grunt!

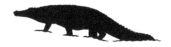

ME: Here (snapping a biscuit in half), share the last biscuit with me, with your coffee.

BEN: Thanks!

9.31 a.m.   A cheerful, large, well-rounded lady delivers a small, square package.

BEN: A little something for you.

ME: Oh (smiling).

BEN: Close your eyes and open your paws.

ME: Okay.

BEN: Open now.

ME: They are *lovely,* and will be nice and light for my weak paws. Thank you!

BEN: I thought you could have fun using them at the beach hut today.

ME: I will!.... It's good that you can order so many things online these days. I feel a song coming on, to the tune of, *I do like to be beside the seaside.*

Oh, I do like it
When you surf a website
And I do like it
When you surf for me
And it's smashing
When you see
Something I'll think
Luverlee

BEN: *Beside the seaside*

ME: *Beside the sea!*

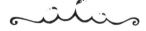

ME: When do you want to set off today?

BEN: Usual time. After the rush hour.

ME: I'll make sure the hairy girls are given their tuna treats, as always, before we go. Keep them happy.

BEN: Bit of a drizzly day.

ME: We'll be cosy in the hut.

BEN: It's gonna get warmer and brighter later.

ME: Oh good.

11.33 a.m.

ME: The decking looks beautiful. Love the colour (stroking the silky woodwork). You've done a *grand job!*

BEN: My pleasure madam.

11.46 a.m.

ME: Guess what? (triumphant grin).

BEN: I can't imagine.

ME: I did it! I actually saved the last four chapters of *The Lighthouse Bookshop* to read today – chapters forty-nine to fifty-three.

BEN: Lots of chapters in that book.

ME: It is a bit doorstep-sized. Nothing like a big, tasty, doorstep book to get your teeth into.

BEN: I fancy one of your doorstep sandwiches now.

ME: I'll pop the whistling kettle on for a cuppa and raid the cool box. We'll have an early lunch. Or late elevenses.

BEN: Late elevenses. Then we can have another lunch.

ME: Good job I packed extra.

BEN: Yeah.

ME: The wind is so chilly and strong, we should have brought hot soup in a flask to warm us up. I've never seen the sea so choppy here.

BEN: We'll be okay with a sandwich in our chops. And we've got the kettle for a hot cuppa.

ME: I'll bring cuppa-soups to store in my lovely, clean cupboards. Bachelors do a delicious broccoli and cauliflower one. And the cream of asparagus is good too, with little crunchy croutons.

1.06 p.m.

ME: Warmer now the sun is out.

BEN: Yeah (tucking into a doorstep-sized cheese and tomato sandwich).

ME: When I've finished these (polishing off a bag of cheese and onion crisps), I think I'll try out my little surprise that arrived today. Can you open the box for me when you've finished your sandwich, it's so firmly and tightly packaged.

BEN: Yep....... open boxes...... take recycling out..... carry shopping...... carry heavy mermaids.

ME: I'm looking forward to bringing Miranda down here.

BEN: Miranda?

ME: My cast iron mermaid. Named after the painting on our bedroom wall by Mr Waterhouse, of a young woman standing on the shore during a storm, watching a ship being wrecked. *Miranda – The Tempest*. When we're next at the hut and the tide is out, I'll take a photo of Miranda in the shallows to send to my niece. She loves mermaids.

BEN: I remember when Louise was little, she was fascinated by our reproduction of *The Mermaid* by Mr Waterhouse. And she thought it was a painting of you, because your hair was very long and the same colour. And the mermaid looks a little like you.

ME: I remember her eyes full of wonder. Bless her.

ME: Oh (giggling), I can see the pier so clearly...... the helter skelter...... row of colourful beach hut shops .... a ship on the horizon... distant seagulls...... and a mermaid! Have a look.

BEN: They are good little binoculars aren't they, nice and light for your paws.

ME: Yes. I used to have some for bird watching, back in the eighties, but they were big and heavy.

BEN: Can't see the mermaid.

ME: You're probably looking in the wrong place. Let me look again.......... that's a shame, she's disappeared. She was naked with, very long, seaweed-brown hair and a beautiful shiny tail (smiling).

BEN: Never mind. I expect only people like you can see mermaids, like you see fairy folk and angels (rolling eyes).... I'll be off for my plod now, and will text you when I'm at the pier. You'll be able to see me with your super, new binoculars. I'll stand on the end of the pier and wave.

ME: I'll watch you waving above the waves. That'll be fun!

BEN: Do you feel some verse coming on about waves and smuggler's caves, and mermaids dancing at seaside raves?

ME: Not at the moment. Have you ever ventured into an old, smugglers cave?

BEN: Nope. Have you?

ME: Yes. Many moons ago. It was at Hastings. I paid for a tour of the caves with friends. I was surprised there were so many small tunnels winding so deep down into the rocks. It was claustrophobic and a little creepy. I recall barrels in corners with soft, spooky lighting.

BEN: Sounds like your perfect day out dear.

ME: It was fun..... I'd like to live in one of those houses, on the Cornish coast that have a secret door, with a tunnel that leads down to a sandy cove, that no doubt was used by smugglers.

BEN: Am I surprised?

1.46 p.m.

ME: Sorry I didn't hear my phone, with all the loud crashing waves. When I checked my phone to see if you'd texted, I saw your message and went out with my binoculars to scan the end of the pier. I peered for quite a while but couldn't see you anywhere at all.

BEN: And I didn't hear your reply. I couldn't stay for long on the pier, it was so cold and windy!

ME: Oh well – next time. On a less cold and windy day.

BEN: Have you finished your book?

ME: Yes. Every last crumb. I'm recalling a quote by Jane Austen:

But for my own part, if a book is well written, I always find it too short.

BEN: Good quote.

ME: True isn't it.

BEN: Yeah.

3.03 p.m.

ME: Did you feel that?!

BEN: What?

ME: An enormous wave crashed onto the pebbles, so close to the hut, it made the floor tremble – wait for the next one.

BEN: Oh yeah, I felt that. The tide must be right in now.

ME: I can hear symbols clashing as trumpets crescendo!

BEN: Really? I can't hear them (looking concerned).

ME: I was listening to Debussy's La Mer this morning on Classic FM. It was a very dramatic piece about waves, wind and the sea. I can still hear it in my head..... Marvellous!

BEN: That's nice (yawning).

3.06 p.m. I wander about twenty feet from the hut, to the end of the first pebbly ridge. Another twenty feet away, an enormous wave splashes onto the shore and I can feel the spray on my face. I breathe in the freshness, smile, then I enjoy a pebbly plod back to the hut.

ME: You'll never guess what I've just seen.

BEN: Surprise me (bigger yawn).

ME: The beautiful mermaid I saw earlier, quite close to the shore. She was swishing her large, silvery-green tail about, and I could feel the spray on my face – very refreshing!

BEN: Did she wave to you?

ME: Yes (smiling).

BEN: Did you wave back?

ME: Of course.

BEN: Fabulous. Pity I missed that (dozing off).

ME: Never mind. Maybe next time.

THE END

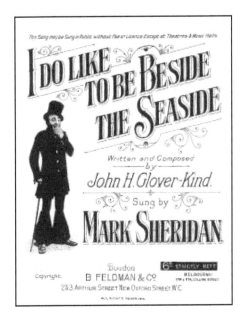

P.T.O

I heard this quote after I had completed my book and put the illustrations in.

It made me cackle so I wanted to put it into the story, but moving the text would move the drawings and spoil the layout.

So I'm popping it in at the end and hope it will make you smile dear reader.

Bread rises in the yeast
And sets in the waist

And as Jim's little grandson Eddie says, this is....

THE REAL END